Praise for Lawrence Kane...

"Lawrence Kane's book, *Martial Arts Instruction*, provides a unique and much-needed professional approach to teaching martial arts. At a time when more and more Americans are seeking personal security through martial arts, Kane's guide to instructors of these ancient skills using modern business and psychological techniques, is incredibly creative and valuable. His practical application of Myers-Briggs personality assessments to students would benefit any teacher, including those training soldiers, security officers, as well as martial artists. Boeing trains hundreds of security officers annually in weapons handling and retention, and Kane's ideas will certainly help us be more effective. The thoughtful discipline he advocates for students and instructors alike, makes this book a must read for anyone seeking to reach the highest levels of martial arts and self defense training." – *Gregory A. Gwash, BA, MA, JD; Chief Security Officer of The Boeing Company; Vietnam Veteran ('65-'67 Special Forces Group).*

"Just because you have your black belt doesn't necessarily mean that you're ready to pass your skills on to others. *Martial Arts Instruction* is a detailed 'how to' book that will be of tremendous value to experienced instructors and novices alike."– *William C. Dietz, author of twenty-five books including the McCade Series, The Drifter Series, The Corvan Series, The Legion Series, and The Sauron Series (Ace Books).*

"*Martial Arts Instruction* is an important text, one that is needed desperately by every instructor and ultimately by every student. Though I've been teaching the martial arts since 1965, I found myself thinking 'I didn't know that' several times as I read this wonderful book. Lawrence A. Kane's research, experience, and writing style make this the definitive work on how to be a better instructor and a better martial artist. Although written primarily for martial arts teachers, I highly recommend this book to all students." – *Loren W. Christensen; martial arts instructor; retired police officer; author of 27 books including Warriors (Paladen) and On Combat, (PPCT Research Publishing) co-authored with Lt. Col. Dave Grossman.*

"This is the book instructors want to have on their desk, and students want their instructors to have open and dog-eared." – *Kris Wilder, martial arts instructor; author of Lessons from the Dojo Floor (Xlibris 2003).*

"Effectively teaching physical combat skills to the variety of students that an average dojo encounters presents difficulties that are not experienced in a normal classroom. Likewise, the average martial arts training in and of itself does not necessarily train one to teach. Lawrence Kane quite effectively clarifies the techniques and skills needed to train the class that a typical instructor will encounter. This is a 'must read' for any new instructor or any instructor that feels he may not be reaching his class." – *Dr. Randall Norstrem, martial arts instructor.*

"His in-depth examination of different personalities provides instructors with an enlightened view of their students and subordinates. His thoughtful and structured techniques lays a foundation and strategy for any class." – *Romadel E. De Las Alas; Lieutenant US Navy; 3-time Iron man Triathlete Finisher.*

"I was a Karate instructor for over twenty years and managed two Karate schools. Lawrence Kane's book is inspiring and a must read for any martial arts instructor. It contains valuable and practical tips for instructors, whether beginning/novice instructors of professional/skilled instructors. The advice on self defense and moral and legal aspects is right on target and sound advice. I would recommend that all martial arts instructors apply the principles Kane identifies to help them become better teachers." – *Vicky M. Peltzer; Police Chief of a Major University; Retired Albuquerque Police Dept. Lieutenant; martial arts instructor.*

"This book is unlike others in that it provides not only teaching content, but also the latest in educational theory to be sure that students receive and make the lessons their own." – *Maureen Kane; Executive Director of Whatcom Literacy Council.*

"I really enjoyed Lawrence's book. It was not only thorough and educational, but also well written and easy to understand. His integration of educational philosophy with the martial arts information gives you not only a visual understanding, but also a deeper appreciation of the art. The use of the Myers Briggs information intertwined with the Japanese training gives the reader a complete understanding of martial arts; it brings together the past with the present. The book is not just a tool for teaching martial arts it can be used as a tool for any teaching situation. It gives solid examples of not only what to teach but how to reach your audience. This book as with the 'core' of martial arts will teach the teacher too." – *Stephen Morissette MA Ed.; Principal of the Holy Family School (Seattle WA).*

"*Martial Arts Instruction* by Lawrence A. Kane provides an outstanding background of teaching Martial Arts through making connections with students' needs, preferences, and learning styles. Mr. Kane's discussions of teaching martial arts are characterized by an extremely well grounded understanding of developmental sequences, learning characteristics and teaching techniques. Reading this text as an educator, I was impressed at the care taken to address the range of abilities and interests of a diverse student population.

"Further, this book provided me with knowledge of an art form and cultural understanding in martial arts that I have had no experience in prior to reading this text. It was engaging, informative, and understandable to read. The examples used placed the reader in an active position mentally to understand the concepts and skills discussed. I want to learn more about the discipline of martial arts as a result of reading this book. I will recommend this book to any student I have who is thinking of studying martial arts or any student that is currently involved with martial arts. It is an excellent reference book." – *Judith A. Perry, Ph. D., M.A.T.; Oregon State University, B.S., National Board for Professional Teaching Standards*

"This book goes beyond its modest stated intention of being about teaching martial arts; it is an insightful guide to good leadership of all kinds. It takes a serious subject and, through a facile mix of theory, practice, and anecdote, leaves the reader feeling empowered to apply its concepts with confidence. Even potentially difficult ideas are so clearly expressed that it is never anything less than lucid. And the jovial, self-deprecating wit and conversational yet authoritative tone is approachable and engaging" – *Bruce A. Ritzen; Attoney-at-Law, Code Reviser and Legislative Drafter.*

"*Martial Arts Instruction* is a winner. Using a variety of powerful tools both traditional and modern, Lawrence Kane has created an impressive roadmap for genuinely passionate martial arts instructors." – *Steven Barnes; author, former Kung Fu columnist for* Black Belt *magazine.*

Martial Arts Instruction

Martial Art
INSTRUCTION

Applying Educational Theory and Communication
Techniques in the Dojo

LAWRENCE A. KANE

YMAA Publication Center
Boston, Mass. USA

YMAA Publication Center, Inc.
Main Office
PO Box 480
Wolfeboro, New Hampshire, 03894
1-800-669-8892 • www.ymaa.com • info@ymaa.com

Edited by Eleanor Sommer
Cover design by Katya Popova
Cover photo courtesy of Punchstock
Text photography by Franco Sanguinetti
Additional photographs courtesy of Kevin Roberts
Tables by the author

ISBN:1-59439-024-x

POD 04512

Publisher's Cataloging in Publication
(Prepared by Quality Books Inc.)

Kane, Lawrence A.
    Martial arts instruction : applying educational theory and
    communication techniques in the dojo / Lawrence A. Kane. -- 1st
    ed. -- Boston, Mass. : YMAA Publication Center, 2004.
        p. ; cm.
        Includes bibliographical references and index.
        ISBN: 1-59439-024-X
        1. Martial arts--Study and teaching. 2. Martial arts--Training.
    3. Educational psychology. 4. Communication in education. I. Title.

GV1102.7.S85 K36 2004   2004112225
796.8/07--dc22   0410

Disclaimer:
The author and publisher of this material are NOT RESPONSIBLE in any manner whatsoever
for any injury which may occur through reading or following the instructions in this manual.
The activities, physical or otherwise, described in this material may be too strenuous or dangerous for some people, and the reader(s) should consult a physician before engaging in them.
Nothing in this document constitutes a legal opinion nor should any of its contents be treated as
such. Questions regarding specific self-defense situations, legal liability, and/or interpretation of
federal, state, or local laws should always be addressed by an attorney.

Printed in USA.

Dedication

For my son Joey, my most important
student in both *budo* and in life.

Table of Contents

Foreword

Upon entering martial arts training, a student can easily recognize the necessity of learning the art. One cannot "scribble" the movements and expect to protect oneself. In fact, the art and the practitioner did not survive or thrive if the art did not work well. Traditional martial arts were honed by the fire of battle. The art and the artist needed to evolve to a high level.

Similarly, in our society, the art of instruction has been developed to high level. Modern psychotherapy, educational research, and scholastic competition have contributed to the enhancement of instructional skills.

However, in our society, martial arts instruction is behind the curve in regards to the "art of instruction." Cross-cultural differences, language difficulties, and rigidness to change have been significant obstacles that we have needed to bridge.

Lawrence Kane is clear and concise in delineating a map to bridge traditional martial arts and modern instructional arts. Students of traditional Japanese martial arts especially will find this book of great use. Be bold, like the author: adapt and adopt ways that will benefit humankind.

I couldn't help but reflect on how I would have benefited from this book when I began teaching martial arts thirty years ago. I was young, presumably adept at martial arts, but woefully inept at teaching. I recognize that this is often the case with many young martial arts teachers. We need this book— and more. Mr. Kane has lit my fire to write. Martial arts instructors need to upgrade their instructional skills to be commensurate with their martial skills. If this can be done, we can bring martial arts to a place of prominence in our society akin to its history in Asia.

Roger Whidden
B.S. in Exercise Physiology
M.A.'s in Education & Therapy
President, Whidden's School of Fitness, Inc.

Preface

"The dojo is a place of awakening, not a hall of competition. The dojo is to be used judiciously to cultivate abilities and to nurture them in their own time, as opposed to demanding progress in technique regardless of circumstance. The dojo is a place to share respect for others, regardless of technical skill... The relationship between student and teacher is complex, based deeply on trust, integrity, and honesty. As a teacher, my duty is to see that the student grows in ability, not because of pressure and competition but in spite of it. As a student, my responsibility is to give my fullest attention to those who would impart something of themselves to bring evolution and well-being to my existence." [1]

– Helen Michiyo Nakano Sensei,
Renshi and co-founder of the
United States Naginata Federation

While the old adage, "those who can't do, teach" is not entirely true, the reverse often enough is. Sadly, "those who can do" frequently cannot teach effectively. As both a student and a teacher I have observed numerous examples of how an educator's actions can encourage or dissuade learning. Through these experiences, I have developed an in-depth understanding of instructional techniques appropriate to a wide variety of situations.

Educators are responsible for employing methodologies that give students productive learning environments where everyone knows what he or she is expected to do and are generally successful at doing it. When the personality mix of the group one is instructing is understood, a teacher may more readily connect with the students' needs, optimizing time and attention to fit individual preferences and learning styles. To achieve the greatest success in effectively communicating with students, educators must be flexible in presentation and approach. One size clearly does not fit all.

In reading this document, martial arts instructors will develop a strategic foundation from which to facilitate student learning and will acquire a discrete toolbox of methods to employ. Educators will improve their abilities to motivate, educate, and retain students, while students will develop a better understanding of what instructional methods best suit their needs.

General subjects covered in this text include the following:

- Understanding the instructional implications of learning style differences
- Using the Myers-Briggs Type Indicator® tool to identify student predilections
- Effectively applying six teaching styles to martial arts instruction
- Fostering an environment conducive to learning
- Developing and implementing lesson plans for the *dojo* (school or training hall) [2]

Teaching martial arts is a fairly serious business. Instructors must balance the somber reality that they are responsible for ensuring the safety of practitioners who learn (potentially) deadly techniques with the truism that if classes are not enjoyable and productive no one will participate. Martial artists are in a unique position to serve as role models for their students whether they intend to or not. Consequently, etiquette and tradition become essential aspects of *budo* (martial ways) training, for without them we would practice nothing more than base violence.

An essential tradition in karate (as with many martial arts) is that practitioners, regardless of rank, bow to each other before practicing together saying, "*Dozo one gaishimasu*" which means, "Please teach me." The implication of this tradition is that teachers will learn from their students as much as students will learn from their instructors. While lower-ranking individuals obviously know less than their more knowledgeable seniors, both parties derive benefit from training together.

Budoka (practitioners of the martial ways) embark upon life-long journeys as they strive to master their chosen arts. A *sensei* (literally, "one who has come before"), or teacher, is simply someone who has progressed further along that path than his or her students. Many martial systems have special ranks to honor highly skilled instructors, especially those who have also excelled in personal and spiritual development. Examples of *shogo*, or teaching titles, include *Hanshi* (model teacher), *Kyoshi* (master teacher), *Renshi* (senior expert), and *Shihan* (expert teacher), all of which recognize exemplary instructors.

By preparing themselves to teach others, *budoka* gain a greater depth of understanding and further the development of themselves and their arts. This is a core concept in all good martial arts: teachers learn from each lesson too.

Acknowledgments

Sincere appreciation to Kris Wilder *Sensei* without whose example this book would never have been written. Special thanks to all my students at the West Seattle Karate Academy. I am honored that you have chosen me for your instructor and want you to know that I learn from you in every class session as well. Heartfelt gratitude to all the people whose knowledge and expertise have honed my *budo* skills and helped me master the art of teaching.

Special thanks to Julieta Kane, David Hsu, and Chuck Friedel who volunteered their time and considerable photographic talents to assist me with the production of this book. The following people modeled for the cameras: Mike Canonica *Sensei*, Duncan Lee, John McNally, Clint Mitchell, Christopher Reilly, Bryan Schenk, Larry Schenk, Maddie Schenk, Scott Schweizer *Sensei*, Jeff Stevens *Sensei*, Michael Thompson, William Thompson, Lindsay Vanderpool, Audrey Vann, Liza Wiberg, Kris Wilder *Sensei*, and Kazel Wood. While not everyone could be included in the limited number of pictures that are published herein, thank you all for giving me part of your weekend.

I would also like to recognize Kevin Roberts *Sensei* who posed for and contributed his *kigu hojo undo* pictures and Franco Sanguinetti *Sensei* who provided pictures of his first-rate *dojo* in San Marcos California. Ellie Sommer deserves special credit for shoring-up my grammatical limitations and otherwise keeping me out of trouble. Thank you one and all!

Introduction

"If you flip through the ads for your local martial arts schools you might get the impression that being some kind of champion is a prerequisite for being an instructor. In reality, what you are is more important than what you have done in the past. To be a good instructor you have to do more than teach. You have to understand and relate to your students. You must have a sense of mission and motivation for what you are doing. You must have knowledge and experience as well as a sense of professionalism. Above all, you have to believe in what you are doing.

"Your teaching method is largely determined by your style, character, cultural-heritage, personality and martial arts background. This means that there can be as many different teaching methods as there are teachers. Still there are fundamental formulas that you can apply to your teaching style to make it as effective as possible." [3]

– *Dr. Sang H. Kim*

In a well-managed *dojo* (or *dojang* in Korean, *kwoon* in Chinese), all students are actively engaged in instructor-led activities or self-directed practice at all times. Not only do they know what they are expected to do, but teaching styles have been thoughtfully selected and communication techniques appropriately tailored such that the students are generally successful. Students feel that they are making progress daily, learning something new, no matter how small, at each training session. There is little to no time wasted due to confusion or disruption. A work-oriented tone prevails, but within a relaxed, pleasant atmosphere.

Children internalize instruction best when it is broken down into simple components. Consequently, complex techniques are best taught as a series of simple movements that, once mastered, can be reintegrated into a whole. While teaching children can be a lot like filling empty vessels with facts and ideas, teaching experienced adults is much more complex. Concepts can no longer simply be poured in; they must be fitted into what is already there. As continuous learners who generally know the modalities by which they learn best (even if they cannot articulate them well), adults gravitate toward instructors whose methods make an effective connection possible.

Instructors who are skilled in identifying learning style and personality type differences can vary their approaches to maximize delivery of their lesson plans in a way that meaningfully connects with their students. Since *budoka* further the development of themselves and their arts when they use these concepts to teach others, one might argue that developing a mastery of teaching is essential to truly mastering any martial art.

An outline of this book's six chapters follows.

Chapter 1: Understanding Learning Style Differences

An understanding of learning-style preferences and personality types greatly facilitates communication between teachers and students. Since different people learn in different ways and process information differently, it is important that educators avoid the common trap of treating students as though they had the same characteristics and preferences as their instructors. Addressing individual learning styles to the extent possible is critical to the success of all class participants.

Physiologically, the five human senses—sight, smell, touch, sound, and taste—are all pathways to the brain. Although students learn in a variety of ways and have a variety of predilections, everyone retains more information when additional neurological pathways are accessed during the learning experience. Keeping this in mind, a good instructor will try to involve as many senses as possible when explaining a new concept. In the martial arts example, an instructor can easily employ demonstration (visual), discussion (auditory), and practice (kinesthetic) in almost any lesson.

Chapter 2: Using the Myers-Briggs Type Indicator® (MBTI®) Tool to Understand Student Predilections

To facilitate communication, world-class educators account for differences in student personality and react accordingly. The MBTI instrument is a widely used personality assessment tool based on Jungian typology, which has proven useful in understanding the role of individual differences in personality type and the implications thereof to the learning process. It is particularly helpful to understand an individual's predilection toward Extraversion or Introversion and his or her inclination toward Sensing or Intuition, two of eight dichotomous dimensions identified by the MBTI tool. This helps instructors understand the degree to which students feel comfortable asking questions and the extent to which the students need to know how and/or why something works before attempting it.

These differences play a significant role in effectively motivating students as well. To be most effective, motivational techniques must be adapted to align with individual student preferences and personality types. In general, however, one can motivate beginners by teaching a variety of simple skills in a straightforward manner while providing regular, positive reinforcement. For intermediate students, instructors should begin to introduce the history and philosophy of their art form and individualize training methods to the extent practicable. For advanced students, instructors should broaden students' knowledge through training and provide opportunities for these more accomplished students to teach others. Personality differences aside, adults tend to be more intrinsically motivated, requiring less handholding than children in educational situations if for no other reason than their basic desire to attend class in the first place.

Chapter 3: Applications of the Six Teaching Styles to Martial Arts

Teachers have a variety of styles available with which they can effectively communicate knowledge. Like tools in a workshop, different teaching styles are appropriate for different applications. The six main teaching styles—modeling, lecturing, cooperative performance, independent performance, knowledge capture, and role reversal—are directly applicable to the instruction of martial arts. Proficient instructors will match each approach to the situation(s) for which it is best suited.

For example, traditional instruction in Asian martial arts relies heavily upon modeling relationships where students observe and attempt to imitate their *sensei's* techniques, transcending potential language barriers and other inhibiters of communication. While this is a particularly powerful method of introducing students to the gross physical movements of an art form, lecturing is required to communicate essential strategic frameworks as well as important nuances of individual tactics or techniques (e.g., stance dynamics, internal power, *sanchin* breathing, or pressure point/nerve manipulation).

Cooperative and independent performance sets in motion a trial and error process through which students develop a better understanding of which techniques are most effective for their unique physical attributes and abilities. Under knowledge capture, the mere process of writing things down facilitates internalization and understanding of the knowledge that is written. By teaching others via role reversal, students internalize the materials taught and develop even deeper understanding.

Chapter 4: Fostering a Positive Learning Environment

The general mindset and biases of the students with whom educators plan to share information will color what they can hear and how they hear it. These biases are both intellectual as well as emotional. Influences on how people will interpret what is presented include their previous experience with and attitude about the subject matter, what is urgent and important to them at the time of instruction, the mental models through which they make sense of the world, any previous experience they might have had (or may have heard about) with the instructor, and any outside issues that may distract their attention.

The instructor's attitude is paramount to effective communication. Martial arts are competency-based, not letter-graded along a curve. When educators truly believe that their primary role is to impart knowledge, they will be motivated to creatively find appropriate mechanisms that ensure their students will learn. Most of the time, when a student does not understand a lesson, it is the teacher's fault.

Etiquette is an integral part of martial arts, for without it we would be practicing nothing more than base violence. Similarly, it is very important to respect the traditions of our art. While boxing, wrestling, and other combat sports are currently associated with name-callers, ear biters, steroid abusers, and generally poor sportsmen (and women), Asian martial arts have managed to maintain their dignity, ostensibly through an adherence to the traditions of such art forms. The primary emphasis of *budo* (martial ways) such as judo, karate, aikido, or kendo is on character development of the *budoka* (*budo* practitioners) themselves rather than on merely training for tournaments or sports competition.

Today, anyone can pay an initiation fee, buy a uniform, and join almost any *dojo* in the country. Few instructors, however, will devote their full attention to new *budoka* until they have proven that they are worthy of such training. The rare student who demonstrates discipline, perseverance, and a positive attitude will gradually be given access to more and more of the instructor's time, attention, and specialized guidance. While all learners deserve a first-rate education, teachers need to be able to recognize and nurture exemplary students just as students need to be able to recognize and adopt excellent instructors.

Chapter 5: Developing and Implementing Lesson Plans for the Dojo

By following a structure of merit, such as the belt system, an instructor has a way of monitoring the development and skill progression of students and can teach them according to set standards. Training objectives must be stated in specific terms so that students will know whether or not these objectives have been met. Continuous feedback is essential in order to assure that students understand how they are progressing. In this fashion, students are able to identify and focus on areas in which they may be deficient. Instructors should monitor student performance over time and promote them once they have met predefined proficiency levels.

Lessons should be approached within a "Plan–Do–Check–Act" framework, allowing for optimal utilization of teacher/student interaction and classroom time management. Under this process, midcourse corrections will ensure that progress is continually achieved and lessons are effectively communicated to the entire student population. Classes should progress through a logical order that both assists in communication and facilitates efficient use of available time. Curricular variety is an important component to maintaining student energy and interest.

Chapter 6: Conclusion/Stages of Teaching

New teachers pass through three relatively distinct developmental phases: induction, consolidation, and mastery. Just as it is essential to understand the personality types and learning styles of students, it is also important to understand the natural progression that teachers follow throughout their careers.

During the induction period, teachers begin to understand how to develop lesson content and present it to their students in an effective manner. In consolidation, teachers refine their understanding to more effectively tailor materials to individual students. On the journey toward mastery, teachers learn through experience and hard work to develop lessons that are enjoyable and beneficial, effective and satisfying for all involved (including themselves). Through long experience and continuing effort, they are able to truly master the art of education, furthering their personal growth, and the development of their martial art.

CHAPTER 1

Understanding Learning
❉ Style Differences ❉

*"Both Higa and Miyagi were very strict and
questions were not permitted during training. When
we practiced, we were not allowed to perform the
kata beyond what they had taught us. In essence you
were not allowed to learn a new sequence of the kata
until the initial section or techniques were
approved... No explanation of techniques was given.
We simply followed instructions. We were not even
permitted to utter a word in response to instructions.
The Sensei often said that they were the "sculptors"
and we were the "raw material" to be sculpted.*

*"Looking back, I realize that teaching the
American GI's really helped me apply Miyagi's theories while developing a cohesive teaching system.
Had I not taught them, my Shorei-kan system would
look nothing like it does today. This may sound con-
fusing, but let me explain. When I taught kata to the
Americans, they always asked questions regarding
the meaning of the kata movements and how they
could be applied to real fighting situations.
Okinawans would never ask such questions."* [4]

– Seikichi Toguchi Sensei

I realized fairly early in life that different people learn and process information in different ways. When teaching and learning styles misalign, students progress slowly, if at all. As a child, I had the opportunity to take judo instruction from a former national champion who was the highest-ranking black belt in the United States at that time. No one could argue that he did not know his art, for truly he had mastered it. Yet in seven years of practice (four years with a three-year break followed by another three years) I truly learned very little, placing no higher than second in a variety of tournament competitions and progressing only to green belt (twice).

In retrospect my natural learning preferences did not properly align with this instructor's teaching style. Similar to the quote about Miyagi *Sensei*, my instructor preferred a traditional modeling approach for instruction (see *Application of the Six Teaching Styles to Martial Arts*) with virtually no explanation or discussion.

While I certainly understood the gross physical movements of each technique he presented, I developed no real understanding of the nuance or subtlety behind what made an individual tactic more or less effective or how it fit into a larger strategy or system. This mismatch not only inhibited my progress but also eventually led me away from judo into the study of other martial forms.

In the early 1980s, I had the opportunity to attend an intensive two-week judo camp taught by a cross-section of instructors. During those two weeks, I experienced enormous variety of teaching styles and methods. Some of these divergent approaches connected with me while others did not. Overall, my skills improved more in those two weeks than they had in all my prior years of training combined.

More importantly, however, I discovered not only which methods worked best for me, but also that what worked well for me was not necessarily the best approach for training other students. This may have been intuitively obvious, but in my prior experience it had never been so aptly demonstrated.

Many years later, I initially approached *Goju Ryu* karate (an Okinawan martial art) with slight trepidation due to my earlier experiences with traditional martial forms. But after sitting in front of a computer for thirteen years, I needed to get into better shape; I hated jogging, was bored with weight lifting, and I wanted to try something new. I found an inexpensive course at a local YMCA and figured it could not hurt to sign-up for a month to give it a try.

Serendipitously, I found an instructor whose teaching approach was able to reach multiple learning styles and was unusually effective at conveying highly complex ideas in easily understandable terms. In fact, his teaching style very closely mirrored the way in which I like to receive information and this greatly facilitated my ability to learn. What began as a one-month trial metamorphosed into several years of training. When he left the YMCA and opened his own *dojo*, I followed him to that location where I continue to train (and teach) today.

Over time, I have found that my instructor is especially adept at making newcomers feel comfortable while maintaining a challenging and interesting curriculum for more advanced students (see *Maintaining Student Interest*). That approach has helped me preserve a high level of interest in *Goju Ryu* and has compelled me to continue my study. He clearly communicates not only nuance and meaning but has also derived modern relevance from traditional technique (see *Tradition*). He also maintains careful control of classroom activities (see *Classroom Management*) and is committed to assuring the safety of his students (see *Physical Environment*), all traits that I find worthy of emulation.

All Students Are Not Alike

"*When all men think alike, no one thinks very much.*" [5]

– *Walter Lippmann*

An understanding of style preferences and personality types greatly facilitates communication between teachers and their students. Addressing individual learning styles to the extent possible is critical to the success of class participants. Instructors must utilize techniques and methodologies that give all students a productive learning environment. Instructors must also avoid the common trap of treating students as though they have the same characteristics and preferences as the instructors themselves do.

Contribution of the Five Senses to Memory Retention

"Memory is the cabinet of imagination, the treasury of reason, the registry of conscience and council chamber of thought." [6]

– Edward M. Forster

Physiologically, the five human senses—sight, smell, touch, sound, and taste—are all pathways to the brain. At the most basic level, people tend to have a primary and secondary pathway preference for processing new information. Any combination of auditory (sound), kinesthetic (touch), and visual (sight) processing preference is possible and will vary by individual. Visual/kinesthetic and auditory/kinesthetic are the most common combinations. While the olfactory sense can trigger a powerful emotional linkage to memory, it is challenging to intentionally incorporate into most instructional situations. Likewise, the sense of taste just isn't used all that much in the teaching of martial arts (or many other subjects outside of culinary arts).

Although different students will have different preferences for their primary learning pathways, all will retain more information when more modes (pathways to the brain) are accessed in the learning experience. Keeping this in mind, good instructors will try to access as many senses as possible throughout instruction, but especially when explaining new concepts or ones with complex or subtle elements. In the martial arts example, instructors can readily employ demonstration (visual), discussion (auditory), and practice (kinesthetic) in an integrated fashion.

Characteristics of Auditory Learners

To teach auditory learners, a martial arts instructor must present information orally, providing specific instructional details such as left/right, front/back, high/low, etc., using Japanese terminology (which is generally more precise than English translations) when appropriate. For Chinese, Korean, Philippine and other martial arts, the language is different but same principle applies. Native language is usually more precise (and pithier) than English translation.

Because such students learn more by hearing or repeating information, they tend to ask lots of questions, often repeating an instructor's answers. Unfortunately, they also have a propensity to want to talk with other students about new techniques rather than physically practicing them. A proper balance must be maintained to assure that auditory learners receive (and discuss when appropriate) reasonably detailed verbal information to facilitate learning while not disrupting classroom flow with idle chatter.

When teaching complicated pattern drills, *kata* (combinations of offensive and defensive techniques done in a particular order), and other combination techniques, I have found it useful to briefly describe each movement just before doing it the first several times it is presented to the class. I might say, for example, "look left, turn, and block left" just before turning in particular stance and executing a left chest block. While these verbal cues do not describe the entire technique, they are enough to help auditory learners to know what to do.

For more advanced students who understand Japanese terminology, the previous example could be stated as, "Look left, turn *zenkutsu dachi*, *chudan hiki uke*." That is a much, much pithier way of saying "look to the left, turn with a sliding crescent step into 'front forward' stance with your front leg bent, back leg straight, legs shoulder width apart, hips and torso aligned, and a 70/30 weight alignment between front and back legs. From there, execute an open hand 'pulling/grasping' chest block keeping your elbows bent, approximately one fist-width away from your body, and closer to your side then your hands, the knuckles of which are held at shoulder height."

It is important to note that instructions given in terms of distance (e.g., inches) will work much more effectively when presented as body lengths (e.g., fist width), as every practitioner will have a different size foot, hand, or arm, etc. In this regard, a standard karate chest block is executed properly when your elbow is one fist width away from your body. Rather than instructing students to step one foot (i.e., twelve inches) forward, it is better to ask them to step forward far enough that the heels of their front feet align with the toes of their back feet.

Characteristics of Kinesthetic Learners

In the *dojo*, kinesthetic learners are probably the easiest students to teach, as they learn primarily by doing. Until such students have practiced a new technique several times they tend to find little value in understanding the concept behind it or the subtleties inherent therein. These students generally find great benefit from exercises practiced with partners. Examples of these include prearranged sequences such as *kiso kumite* (presequenced sparring) or *kata bunkai* (applications from *kata*).

Unfortunately, kinesthetic learners often have trouble staying still, a trait that could be interpreted as not paying attention even when they are completely focused on the instructor. They also have a propensity to copy instructor's demonstrations in attempts to internalize new lessons, another habit that could be misinterpreted as a lack of respect. For the most part, fidgeting by kinesthetic learners should be ignored (so long as it is not disruptive to other students).

As they struggle to learn new skills, I frequently "freeze" the class then go around and physically move students into correct body alignment for a given technique. For example, if someone's chest block is too far to the outside, the elbow is not closer to the body than the fist, or the person's posture is otherwise incorrect, I will move the arm into the proper place.

Once it is in the proper position, I will press against it for a moment so that the student can feel the strength of correct technique, then I'll move it back into the previous improper configuration and apply pressure. Finally, I will replace the arm

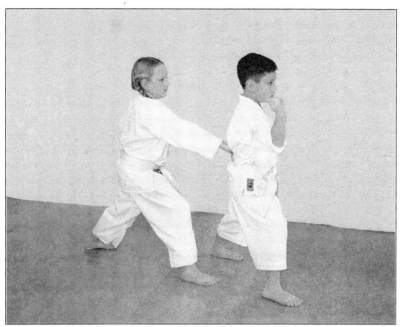

IN THE TANDEM DRILL PICTURED HERE, ONE PRACTITIONER MOVES FORWARD IN *ZENKUTSU DACHI* (FRONT FORWARD STANCE) WHILE THE OTHER OFFERS RESISTANCE BY HOLDING HIS BELT. SUCH MANEUVERS REINFORCE PROPER BODY MECHANICS AND BALANCE, ACCLIMATIZING KINESTHETIC LEARNERS TO THE STANCE.[A]

where it belongs, pressing against it a final time. In this manner, kinesthetic learners can understand the "feel" of doing movements properly, internalizing which positions are weak and which are strong. Misalignment by a mere half inch may mean the difference between brutally effective and hopelessly ineffectual technique. Such minor nuances can often be felt even when they cannot readily be seen.

When teaching complicated pattern drills, *kata*, and other combination techniques for the first time, I have found it useful to train together as a group until students understand the basic pattern and then let them continue at their own paces under the tutelage of a senior student. That allows me to watch and make corrections on an individual basis by "freezing" people and realigning their postures until they are correct.

Characteristics of Visual Learners

In order to understand new information, visual learners must clearly see demonstrations. In the *dojo*, it is important to intersperse senior and junior students during moving drills or *kata* such that visual learners can see and emulate technique from whichever direction they are facing. Mirrored walls are an excellent addition to the *dojo* because they facilitate improvement for all students, especially visual learners. Visual learners also benefit from supplemental reading materials, web sites, and/or videotapes. Therefore, an instructor can reinforce learning by providing reading lists or handouts, promoting the use of journals or notebooks, or even by drawing diagrams on a whiteboard.

Some *dojos* maintain a library of books and/or videos that students can utilize to supplement their classroom training. We have a comprehensive set of notes that students are encouraged to copy if they are interested. Many instructors videotape *kata* practice and sparring sessions so that visual learners can objec-

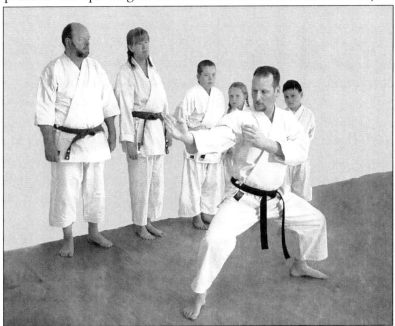

SENSEI DEMONSTRATES *SAIPAI* WHILE THE CLASS OBSERVES THE *KATA*. VISUAL LEARNERS BENEFIT FROM WATCHING TECHNIQUES BEFORE ATTEMPTING TO DO THEM ON THEIR OWN.[B]

tively evaluate their performances after the fact and receive appropriate coaching for improvement (sort of like reviewing game films in football).

When teaching complicated pattern drills, *kata*, and other combination techniques for the first time, I have found it useful to draw the pattern on a white board and demonstrate all of the movements to the class before having them follow along. I then break it down into small pieces that everyone can practice together. I ensure that senior and junior students are interspersed, of course, so that no matter what direction we are facing everyone can see someone to imitate. Each time there is a direction shift, I briefly pause everyone's movement while I reposition myself in front of the group so that all students can easily see what I am doing as well.

Summary

An understanding of learning-style preferences and personality types greatly facilitates communication between teachers and their students. Since different people learn in different ways and process information differently, it is important that an educator avoid the common trap of treating students as though they had the same characteristics and preferences as the instructor does. Addressing individual learning styles to the extent possible is critical to the success of all class participants.

Physiologically, the five human senses—sight, smell, touch, sound, and taste—are all pathways to the brain. Although there is great variety in student mode predilections, everyone will retain more information as additional pathways are accessed during the learning experience. Keeping this in mind, a good instructor will try to involve as many senses as possible when explaining a new concept.

The following briefly summarizes how best to teach to the three main senses discussed previously:

To teach auditory learners, a martial arts instructor must present information orally, providing specific instructional details such as left/right, front/back, high/low, etc. Reasonable efforts should be made to include Japanese terminology, which is generally more precise than English translations.

Tandem drills and repetition are especially beneficial for kinesthetic learners who gain skills primarily by doing.

Because visual learners must clearly see demonstrations, it is important to intersperse senior and junior students such that everyone can see and emulate proper technique from whichever direction they are facing.

To help everyone at once, instructors should strive to employ demonstration (visual), discussion (auditory), and practice (kinesthetic) in each lesson.

CHAPTER 2

Using the Myers-Briggs Type Indicator® (MBTI®) Tool to Understand ☀ Student Predilections ☀

"The MBTI was developed by the mother and daughter combination of Isabel Myers and Katherine Briggs in an effort to operationalize the theories of renowned psychiatrist Karl Jung. It was used successfully during World War II in placing civilians in jobs required by the war effort. It has since been revised several times and is constantly being tested for validity and reliability." [7]

– Paladin Associates, a consulting group

The Myers-Briggs Type Indicator (MBTI) is a useful tool to help educators understand the role of individual differences in personality type and implications thereof to the learning process. Scores obtained from the MBTI indicate a person's preference on each of four dichotomous dimensions, leading to sixteen categories or personality type combinations. These dimensions include Extraversion (E) or Introversion (I), Intuition (N) or Sensing (S), Thinking (T) or Feeling (F), and Perceiving (P) or Judging (J).

Myers-Briggs Type Indicator

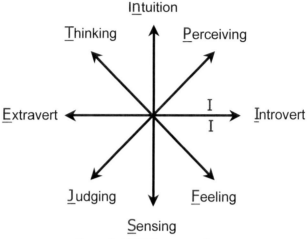

FIGURE 1. MBTI DIMENSIONS CHART

Understanding Personality Types

"You see things as they are and ask, why? I dream things as they never were and ask, why not?" [8]

– George Bernard Shaw

By understanding the personality mix of the group he or she is instructing, an educator may more readily connect with the students' needs, optimizing time and attention to fit their preferences and individual learning styles. One size clearly does not fit all. To achieve the greatest success in effectively communicating with students, educators need to be flexible in presentation and approach.

Table 1 describes all sixteen MBTI personality type combinations. The number in parenthesis represents the approximate percentage of the population that displays each preference. A review of this table highlights differences and similarities between personality types.

Educators who thoroughly understand MBTI characteris-

		Sensing Types		Intuitive Types	
		With Thinking	With Feeling	With Feeling	With Thinking
Introverts	Judging	ISTJ (6%) "Investigator" – Serious, quiet, well organized and thorough. Achieves through steady progression toward goal regardless of distraction. Fine motor skilled.	ISFJ (6%) "Assistant" – Responsible, accurate detailed, patient and conscientious. Often needs time to master technical subjects. Gross motor skilled.	INFJ (1%) "Wordsmith" – Firmly principled. Puts best effort into work, achieving through perseverance, originality, and desire. Language skilled.	INTJ (1%) "Inventor" – Skeptical, critical, original, independent, and determined. Work hard in areas of personal interested. Logical abstraction skilled.
	Perceptive	ISTP (5%) "Athlete" – Quiet, reserved, analytical, and detached. Artful with tools and hands. Exerts no more effort than thinks necessary. Fine motor skilled.	ISFP (5%) "Artisan" – Quiet, friendly, sensitive. Shuns disagreements. Enjoys the present moment avoiding undue haste or exertion. Gross motor skilled.	INFP (1%) "Idealist" – Quiet until he/she knows you. Works hard and independently, but frequently too absorbed tasks to be sociable. Language skilled.	INTP (1%) "Logician" – Logical to the point of hair-splitting. Interested mainly in big ideas and theoretical subjects while avoiding small talk. Logical abstraction skilled.
Extraverts	Perceptive	ESTP (13%) "Opportunist" – Matter of fact; lives in present. Tends to focus on mechanical things and sports. Dislikes long or detailed explanations. Fine motor skilled.	ESFP (15%) "Entertainer" – Sound common sense and practical ability with people as well as things. Remembers facts easier than mastering theories. Gross motor skilled.	ENFP (5%) "Motivator" – Enthusiastic, innovative, and imaginative. Often relies on ability to improvise rather than preparing in advance. Language skilled.	ENTP (5%) "Strategizer" – Outspoken, logical, and often argumentative. Resourceful in solving new challenges but quickly tires of routine. Logical abstraction skilled.
	Judging	ESTJ (13%) "Supervisor" – Practical realist. Likes to organize and run things. Not interested in subjects for which he/she sees no practical use. Fine motor skilled.	ESFJ (13%) "Facilitator" – Warm-hearted, talkative, cooperative, and teaming. Little interest in abstract thinking or technical subjects. Gross motor skilled.	ENFJ (5%) "Educator" – Leads with ease and tact, demonstrating concern for others. Able to balance priorities and complete quality work. Language skilled.	ENTJ (5%) "CEO" – Frank, strong-willed. Good at reasoning and public speaking but often more confident than knowledgeable. Logical abstraction skilled.

TABLE 1. MBTI PERSONALITY TYPE COMBINATIONS.

tics can tailor their teaching methodologies to ensure compatibility with student preferences. It should be noted, however, that while it is impossible accommodate all styles simultaneously, it is nevertheless important to understand all of them. See *Accommodating Learning Style Preferences* for a discussion on how to focus on the subset of characteristics that facilitates meaningful tailoring of educational technique.

Extraversion (E)

Successful strategies for teaching Extraverts generally include interactive assignments using collaborative work groups, freeform discussions, or spirited debates to exchange information and stimulate learning. When it comes to assignments, these individuals often prefer to present coursework orally rather than in a written fashion.

Introversion (I)

For Introverts, instructors should integrate and connect subject matter, teaching in logical chunks of interconnected facts. It is often useful to help such students develop their own frameworks for learning where practical. These individuals generally prefer to think and reflect on coursework, typically excelling at written assignments while being challenged by interactive discussions. When debate is required, an effective method of meliorating this difficulty is to allow sufficient "think" time for Introverts to deliberate prior to the commencement of any verbal interchange.

Intuition (N)
Intuitive students like more generalized concept maps and learn well using a "theory–application–theory" approach. These individuals are comfortable working with hunches and other unexplainable ways of knowing, looking for patterns, meanings, and future possibilities. While they excel at creative coursework, they are often bored by, and resistant to, routine assignments. Curricular variety is essential.

Sensing (S)
Successful strategies for teaching Sensing students include organized, linear, structured lessons conducted in an "application–theory–application" approach. Such students appreciate early understanding of instructional objectives so that they can prepare for what they must know in advance. They prefer to work with "givens" in the "real world" rather than with abstract theories or possibilities.

Thinking (T)
Thinking students generally focus on facts and data. They strongly believe in, and generally want to comply with, objectives, principles, and policies. They have a strong preference for organizing and structuring information in logical, objective ways. Successful strategies for such students include ensuring clearly defined and documented course objectives with precise, action-oriented assignments. Instructors should always be clear and unambiguous when communicating with these students.

Feeling (F)

Feeling students tend to be subjective, values-based individuals, who focus on emotion rather than fact. They have preferences for organizing and structuring information in a personal, value-oriented ways. Successful strategies for teaching such students include interactive group activities, open discussions, and harmonious social interactions.

Perceiving (P)

Because individuals who prefer Perceiving are flexible and open to experience, they often have many things going on at once. Successful strategies for such students include breaking assignments into small steps with interim deadlines to assure completion. These individuals excel in situations that allow for spontaneity and creativity.

Judging (J)

Students who prefer Judging like to analyze, organize, and respond, often testing conventional theory. They are goal oriented and enjoy situations that are organized and scheduled. Instructors who play the "devil's advocate" and encourage reverse questioning or debate are often appreciated. Lessons for such individuals should be well structured with activities and timeframes prearranged.

Strengths by MBTI Type

Although the aforementioned preferences could appear, at first blush, to add value primarily in the realm of academia, an understanding of these differences can help all educators, including those who teach physical activities such as martial arts. In addition to their learning style preferences, each student will also have a predisposition to excel in various areas based on his/her personality type. Martial arts students must be taught in ways that extenuate their strengths while minimizing their weaknesses.

Sensing Thinking (ST) personality types tend to develop fine motor skills, while Sensing Feeling (SF) types are more adept at gross motor skills. Intuitive Feeling (NF) types have an affinity for language skills while Intuitive Thinking (NT) personalities excel at logical abstraction.

Determining your MBTI Type

Determining MBTI type for the purpose of understanding personality differences within a work group has frequently been used as a team-building exercise in Fortune 500 companies such as Boeing. A part-time karate instructor, I actually earn my living as a financial analyst for the Boeing Company. When I interviewed for my current position, my perspective boss and I discussed our personality types during the interview. It was very helpful in setting expectations and has allowed me to perform better once I got the job.

Answers to MBTI questions are scored and sorted on either side of scale so that there are varying degrees of clarity to whatever preference is indicated. While I am very clear that I am an E on the E–I scale, for example, I am less clear about my S–N preference. My boss, like most other executives I work with both inside and outside the company, is a Promethean personality (*see Four Temperaments*) with very clear NT preferences: specifically he is an ENTJ.

By understanding my boss's personality type, I can tailor my approach to communicate with him more effectively. Tailoring should never be confused with "sucking up" or selling out. While I may modify presentations or conversations to meet his preferences, I still complete my work in the way in which I perform best. I still think and do things in my own way. I simply communicate more effectively by approaching different people in a manner that meets their individual preferences. The same principle applies in teacher/student relations, of course.

Promethean (NT) personalities, especially corporate executives with NT personalities, really want to know the "bottom line" before worrying about details. Approaching such individuals in an inductive manner by presenting the *answer* first works best. My boss has no patience for deductive conversations that belatedly arrive at a conclusion. Another important implication of ENTJ individuals is that they generally want to "do" things or "fix" things when presented a problem. I am always careful to let my boss know up front whether I will simply be giving him the status on something or if I'm asking him for help. This reduces tension and minimizes confusion very effectively. And, I'm less likely to get "help" when I don't really need (or want) it.

Martial arts instructors often have bosses too. It is certainly safe to assume that they have students. Although an MBTI exercise could be arranged for a *dojo* just as easily as it could be completed at a corporation, it is much less regularly done in that venue. By careful observation, however, instructors can often ascertain their students' personality traits (*see Applying MBTI to Accommodate Student Predilections*), even when the students themselves cannot or will not articulate them effectively.

No matter how well you know yourself, it can be hard to adequately express your predilections without a structured approach like the MBTI tool. Many consultants and professional resources (such as www.keirsey.com, www.advisorteam.com, or www.capt.org) are available to help individuals ascertain and understand their personality types in more depth than can be covered here.

Since a large number of colleges, private companies, and large corporations incorporate such testing into their placement, development, and/or training processes, many readers will already know their MBTI types. If you do not know MBTI type, you can use a simple test that I have devised to help you make an educated guess about your preferences. While only the official MBTI instrument can determine a person's *MBTI type*, there are many clues to your psychological type. Ultimately, even when you take the MBTI instrument, the test itself is used as an indication not as a determination; each person is required to verify his or her type based on their own experience, even when that choice differs from the scored results of the MBTI instrument. (See appendix C—Determining Your Psychological Type).

Accommodating Learning Style Preferences

"When mismatches exist between learning styles of most students in a class and the teaching style of the professor, the students may become bored and inattentive in class, do poorly on tests, get discouraged about the courses, the curriculum, and themselves, and in some cases change to other curricula or drop out of school. Professors, confronted by low test grades, unresponsive or hostile classes, poor attendance and dropouts, know something is not working. They may become overly critical of their students (making things even worse) or begin to wonder if they are in the right profession. Most seriously, society loses potentially excellent professionals." [9]

– Dr. Richard M. Felder, Professor Emeritus of Chemical Engineering, North Carolina State University

Understanding the sixteen MBTI types in sufficient detail to develop course curriculum can be a particularly daunting task. Obviously catering to multiple, divergent personality preference combinations at the same time would result in dichotomous, unrealistic teaching methods—all the personalities clearly cannot all be accommodated simultaneously. It is simpler (and more practical), yet still quite useful to focus on a subset of these dimensions, two of which are particularly helpful in understanding learning-style preferences:

- Extraversion (E) or Introversion (I)
- Sensing (S) or Intuition (N)

Extraversion–Introversion indicates whether a person prefers to direct attention toward the external world of people and things or toward the inner world of concepts and ideas. The Sensing–Intuition dichotomy indicates whether a person prefers perceiving the world through directly observing the surrounding tangible reality or through impressions and imagined possibilities.

Characteristics of Extraverts or Introverts

Extraverted people draw energy from outside themselves, thriving on interactions with people, activities, and things. As students, they tend to be action oriented, learning well in a "do–think–do" environment. They actively participate, ask questions, and get involved in the learning process. An inherent strength of this personality type is that instructors immediately know when Extraverts need additional understanding or are confused about a lesson or instruction. Be aware though that Extraverts have a tendency to monopolize a teacher's attention by asking a disproportional number of questions or engaging in prolonged discussions.

Introverted people draw energy from their internal world of ideas, emotions, and impressions. As students they tend to be reflection oriented, learning best in a "think–do–think" environment. Even when they are thoroughly engaged in the learning process, they may appear too distant, distracted, or a step behind the other students. Introverts are often uncomfortable asking for help and must sometimes be actively drawn into conversations.

A prudent educator will balance maintaining enthusiasm and participation from Extraverts with actively engaging reticent Introverts whose needs might easily be overlooked.

Characteristics of Sensing or Intuition

In general, students who prefer Sensing learning patterns naturally gravitate toward the practical and the immediate. Their learning styles are characterized by a preference for direct, concrete experiences, moderate to high degrees of structure, linear or sequential learning, and a need to know *why* before doing something. They are often less independent in thought and judgment and may require frequent coaching or direct instruction.

Intuitive individuals are generally "big picture" types who prefer to focus on imaginative possibilities rather than on concrete realities. This personality type likes to move from theory to practice, typically disliking the highly structured learning environments that work well for Sensing individuals. They can more readily accommodate ambiguity, usually demonstrating a high degree of autonomy in their learning, and valuing knowledge for its own sake. These individuals are often more independent and require less frequent coaching or direct instruction.

A wise educator will oversee student activities in a manner compatible with the level of autonomy and structure that facilitates achievement. This often requires tailoring to some degree to accommodate individual style preferences. When you accurately understand each student's preferences between Sensing and Intuition, you can spend more time with some students without causing others to feel left out.

For example, Intuitive types can be afforded "open" *dojo* time to work on their advancement requirements while individuals with a Sensing preference can simultaneously perform structured drills that cover what they need to know. If you are not certain who fits into what category, you can always let students choose which group (e.g., open *dojo* or group *kata*) they would like to join, and they will generally sort themselves out for you.

Observable Behavior Patterns

"Odd about humans: they've been trying to categorize and understand themselves ever since ever. Know what? When it comes to personalities, almost every philosophizer has decided on four dominant types. For Hippocrates it was Sanguine, Choleric, Phlegmatic and Melancholic. Jung decided on Feeler, Thinker, Sensor and Intuitor. Keirsey calls them Idealists, Rationals, Guardians and Artisans." [10]

– Future Now, a consulting group

Myers-Briggs Type	Temperament	Preferred Learning Style	Preferred Work Style	Natural Leadership Style	Known For Contributing
SJ	Epimethean – organizer, stabilizer	Step-by-step with preparation for current and future utility	Responsibility, loyalty, and industry	Traditionalist, stabilizer, consolidator	Timely output
SP	Dionysian – negotiator, troubleshooter	Through active involvement to meet current needs	Action, cleverness, and timeliness	Troubleshooter, negotiator, fire fighter	Expeditious handling of the unexpected
NF	Apollonian – catalyst, team builder	For self awareness through personalized and imaginative ways	People, values and inspirations	Catalyst, spokesperson, energizer	Personal or special vision of possibilities
NT	Promethean – creator, visionary	Impersonal and analytical process for personal mastery	Ideas, ingenuity, and logic	Visionary, architect, builder	Strategies and analysis

TABLE 2. FOUR TEMPERAMENTS.

Another practical way of grouping personality preferences is based on observable behavior patterns or *temperaments*. As far back as ancient Greek times, these temperaments have historically been used to describe differences between people in a manner that is relatively easy to grasp. These descriptions are particularly valuable when attempting to understand and accommodate learning style preferences.

Applying MBTI to Accommodate Student Predilections

"Softness triumphs over hardness, feebleness over strength. What is more malleable is always superior over that which is immovable. This is the principle of controlling things by going along with them, of mastery through adaptation." [11]

– Lao Tzu

A good understanding of MBTI principles gives instructors added flexibility in understanding and dealing with student personality differences. As with anything, the more practice one has in applying these concepts the easier it becomes. If I don't already know someone's personality type, I attempt to figure it out as practically and expeditiously as I can. With this goal in mind, I tend to focus on two areas: (1) Introversion or Extraversion and (2) Sensing or Intuition, which I blend with the concepts of auditory, visual, and kinesthetic learning to rapidly identify and classify my students and to form individually effective teaching strategies for each. This can be a very powerful methodology for discovering how to accommodate student preferences.

In general, it is usually okay to assume someone's preferences, but it is prudent to confirm that you are correct before taking any action. Determining whether someone is extroverted or introverted is almost always readily apparent once you have been around him or her for a short time. Sensing or Intuition, on the other hand, is somewhat more problematic. By exercising active listening skills (see *How to be an Active Listener*) and asking probing questions, I have found that it is possible to rapidly ascertain whether someone prefers a Sensing or Intuitive approach. Regardless of whether I know a student's preferred learning mode, I try to teach to auditory, visual, and kinesthetic preferences in every lesson.

While I was writing this book, a new student enrolled in the *dojo*. She is a well-educated attorney who is in her late 30s or early 40s and very athletic and in excellent shape. She appeared highly motivated to learn a martial art. She was clearly introverted and said almost nothing to her fellow students or teachers before, during, or after class. Although she tackled the lessons with great intensity, after just a couple of sessions her body language made it readily apparent that she was getting more and more frustrated as the day wore on. Unfortunately she left too quickly after the class for me to find out why.

When she arrived a couple of minutes early for a subsequent class, I made a point of asking her how the training was going and whether or not she was enjoying the class. Although her initial response indicated that everything was fine, her body language told a different story. I probed gently, asking open-ended questions and listening attentively until she admitted her frustration. She had developed very high expectations for herself, in my mind unrealistically so. Because of this she was quite upset that she could not perform techniques as well as other people in the class. I gathered that she had a long history of easily succeeding in all her endeavors throughout her prior academic and professional life.

If I told her that everyone else in the class had been training at least two months longer than she had, it may have been illuminating, perhaps, but hardly helpful. Explaining that all new students struggle for the first few months would clearly not have been an appropriate answer either, as it would most likely have come across as an insincere brush-off. Suggesting that she train outside of class would also have been unhelpful as she had already told me that she was afraid of learning something incorrectly and having to turn-around and unlearn it again. This was a bit of a quandary, and I felt that I had only one opportunity to figure out how to respond affectively, as she appeared ready to quit.

As I mentioned, the fact that she was introverted was quite obvious. Based on her background and one short conversation, I surmised that she was most likely a Sensing type personality, someone who likes a lot of structure, thinks fairly linearly, and wants to understand things before doing them. I intuited this primarily based on her comments regarding reluctance to practice outside of class. Speculating that she might also be a visual learner (lawyers have to read a lot and people frequently gravitate toward professions that fit their predilections), I asked if she thought that supplemental reading materials might help.

This was clearly a guess on my part, although a reasonably educated one. I determined, however, that there was very little downside in asking. When queried in this manner she affirmed my supposition, indicating that reading materials would be very welcome. I recommended a couple of books on *Goju Ryu;* ones that I believed explained the basic techniques and initial *katas* with thorough enough descriptions to help a beginner without being overwhelming. I specifically selected ones with well-done photographs and graphics. I also promised to give her a copy of some notes I had compiled (something we encourage students to use anyway). The notes, a compilation of my personal scribblings over the years, explain many of the things she was struggling to learn, though they are almost entirely text and do not stand alone well without instructional support.

Anticipation of receiving this supplemental information seemed to keep her motivated through that day's class. She seemed even more positive during the following week. My advice was certainly not a panacea, but it clearly hit the target in making her feel better about the training. Not only was she appreciative of my suggestions but I also saw marked improvement in her execution of the techniques over the next several sessions. Later on she mentioned that the written materials helped her feel comfortable performing solo training outside of class, as she could be certain that she was practicing the techniques correctly.

There is another individual who has been attending our *dojo* for a couple of years now. He is very similar to the aforementioned attorney in that he is also highly educated (an MBA), approximately the same age, very athletic, and also great shape. He really loves karate, driving more than twenty miles through Seattle traffic (some of the worst in the nation) to attend class. His preferences, however, are quite different.

A fellow Introvert and perfectionist who sets challenging goals for himself, he is nevertheless an Intuitive. He also has a strong penchant for kinesthetic learning. This combination makes him very fervently prefer to practice techniques numerous times before learning how they fit into the strategic context or why they are done in the way they are shown. He certainly feels that such things are important, just not right at the beginning.

Since I have a propensity to over-explain things in his mind, and under-explain them in the minds of others (like the aforementioned attorney), I have had to form a strategy that keeps everyone happy (to the extent possible, of course). When working with the entire class, I tend to offer minimal explanations of basic forms or activities that most people have seen before. When teaching something new, I may offer a bit more explanation (e.g., drawing the pattern on a white board or explaining how a technique fits into the strategy of *Goju Ryu*), but generally I let the group work through the material a few times before going into more depth. After this initial introduction, however, I break students into smaller groups to refine what they are learning.

Frequently I will consciously try to keep the Intuitive individuals and Sensing individuals separated. By ensuring that students are grouped with others of similar ilk, they are able to train in a manner that best suits their styles. In this fashion, I am able to accommodate dichotomous preferences simultaneously. I do not exclusively employ this approach, however, as diversity is an important component of learning as well and disparate personality types will often help each other understand their blind spots and exceed their own limitations.

How to be an Active Listener:
Active listening is a great tool for deciphering student personality types and learning their predilections. It also demonstrates respect for students and interest in their issues. Whenever possible, instructors should strive to exercise active listening skills, especially when interacting with adult learners.

An ancient Native American tradition called the "talking stick" or talking stick circle was an important ritual at gatherings, where a decorated stick was passed around to those who wished to speak (bringing a piece of truth into the circle). Only the person holding the stick was allowed to talk at any given time (hence the name). This kept cross talk and disruption to a minimum.

The most interesting part of this tradition centered on times when someone wished to dispute another person's opinion. Before contradicting someone else's statement, you had to express his or her perspective using your own words until the person was satisfied that you understood his or her point of view. Only after reaching that stage could you disagree. This tradition is an outstanding example of active listening.

Teachers can listen actively by using the following methods:

- Remaining neutral to the extent possible.
- Giving complete attention.
- Asking clarifying questions.
- Restating the student's main points as necessary to clarify understanding.

Remaining neutral is often harder than it sounds. In conversations many people do not really listen to what others are saying because they are busy formulating their own responses or thinking up better ways to explain their own perspectives. As demonstrated by the talking stick ritual, it is far better to understand the other party first. Only then should you seek to be understood, presenting your own perspective.

Giving complete attention is also easier said than done. This means focusing only on the student to whom you are listening, ignoring all but life-threatening distractions. Since a significant part of communication comes from nonverbal cues, pay attention to your body language. Maintain direct eye contact, lean slightly forward, and resist any desire to fidget (especially if you are a kinesthetic learner).

The concept of asking clarifying questions is fairly self-evident, but there is an art to doing it right. You queries should be used to subtly demonstrate understanding and sympathy for the student's perspective. That does not mean that you have to agree, merely understand.

Restating the student's main points, as necessary, is an excellent way to clarify understanding. Like the talking stick ritual, this is a very positive way of ensuring that you really understand where a student is coming from. By restating the points in your own words, you can be supportive of the students as individuals whether or not you agree with the particular opinions they expressed. Active listening demonstrates respect for a student's perspective and can also be very motivational as well.

Applying MBTI Preferences to Motivate Martial Arts Students

"Walk a single path, becoming neither cocky with victory nor broken with defeat, without forgetting caution when all is quiet or becoming frightened when danger threatens." [12]

– *Professor Jigoro Kano Sensei,*
founder of Kodokan Judo

World-class educators account for differences in student personalities and react accordingly to facilitate communication. As was outlined above, some students are comfortable working independently while others require more rigid structure. Some students need to understand why something works before attempting it, while others are happy to jump right in and perform. These differences also play a significant role in effectively motivating students. To be most effective, motivational techniques must be adapted to align with individual preferences and personality types of the students.

Learning martial arts can truly be a life changing experience. In addition to the obvious fitness and self-defense benefits, the impact to a student's self-esteem is often profound. It could be a seemingly inconsequential event such as a shy, quiet kid letting out a really strong, loud *kiai* (shout) for the first time, or something more significant such as when that same child finds the inner confidence to lead the entire class in *kata*. Through these events, a student's sense of self-worth is measurably improved. This is not only true for Introverts, but for Extraverts as well. When Extraverts progress, however, the impact on their self-esteem is not as readily observable.

Some students are *intrinsically* motivated while others are *extrinsically* motivated. Internally motivated individuals will typically rise to challenges. If, for example, these personality types are promoted before they think they are ready, it will be taken as a challenge to work harder. Extrinsically motivated individuals, on the other hand, might harbor resentment if they see others around them being promoted and feel that they have been passed over. Consequently, motivational techniques must be tailored to the individual to the extent possible (see *Testing and Advancement Principles*).

For some, a word of praise is beneficial, yet for others it is required. While some traditionalist-minded instructors may assume that compliments automatically lead to laziness and that all students should be intrinsically motivated, I believe that American psyche requires a certain level of regular positive feedback. Praise is an interesting thing, however. No matter how well intentioned, generalized praise can backfire, being seen as halfhearted at best and condescending or backhanded at worst. Always be specific.

Rather than saying, "[Name], you did real well tonight," for example, instructors should specifically identify what noteworthy accomplishments the student made (e.g., paying better attention; trying harder; and/or specific technique, such as stance, movement, breathing, punching, kicking, blocking, and so on). While public praise is especially beneficial for extrinsically motivated individuals, it is valuable for all students.

Ensure continuous student motivation by establishing personal contact, actively engaging students in the learning process, ensuring that feedback is constructive and specific, creating an environment where participants feel comfortable asking questions, and tailoring the educational approach to meet participant learning style preferences. Above all, instructors must remain fair and impartial in the treatment of all students.

Certain distinctions exist between effective methods of motivating children and methods for encouraging adults. Personality differences aside, adults are more often intrinsically motivated, requiring less handholding than children in educational situations.

Children, who are often forced into educational situations by their parents, generally need more active encouragement, patience, and understanding than adults who attend voluntarily. Frequent feedback, a variety of activities, and positive reinforcement are essential for connecting with youth in these situations. For younger students, praise in front of their peers and/or parents is particularly motivational.

Maintaining Student Interest

Even those with the best initial attitude working in the most positive and supportive environments will eventually reach plateaus in their training, working for long periods of time without the perception of improvement. When practitioners feel stymied and struggle to make progress, they are frequently inclined to abandon their training. This may be part of the reason why so many practitioners drop out in the middle

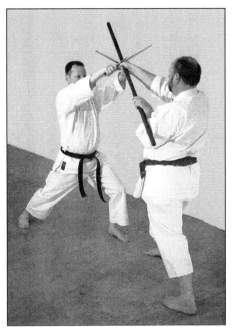

MATAYOSHI *KOBUDO* UTILIZES MANY OF THE SAME STANCES AND BODY MECHANICS AS *GOJU RYU* KARATE. IN THIS FASHION, WEAPONS FORMS CAN SUPPLEMENT OPEN-HANDED MARTIAL WAYS, OFFERING IMPORTANT PERSPECTIVES IN AREAS THAT OVERLAP. VARIETY IS A GOOD WAY TO KEEP STUDENTS MOTIVATED AND ENGAGED SO LONG AS IT FITS WITHIN AN OVERALL CURRICU-LUM AND DOES NOT BECOME OVERWHELMING.[C]

ranks and why a large number of others do so after attaining their first-degree black belt. In many systems the skill differential between first- and second-degree is humongous (similar to the gap between a white belt and a black belt). Once practitioners truly understand the magnitude of that gap they may become discouraged, deciding that it takes too much effort to bridge it. During these times it is especially important for instructors to provide ongoing extrinsic motivation.

Variety is also important. Even though my current *sensei* is an excellent teacher, I have reached important epiphanies and broken through plateaus in my training after experiencing another instructor or student's perspective. Inviting guests to teach a class or seminar on occasion can broaden students' education and help maintain their interest. Students and teachers

1) Beginners
   a) Begin with a variety of simple skills
   b) Teach in a straightforward manner
   c) Provide positive reinforcement
2) Intermediate
   a) Introduce history and philosophy
   b) Individualize training methods
   c) Increase intrinsic motivation by minimizing feedback
3) Advanced
   a) Broaden knowledge through instructor training
   b) Encourage perfection of skills and self-fulfillment
   c) Provide opportunities to teach

FIGURE 2.1. MAINTAINING STUDENT INTEREST.

alike can benefit from exposure to a variety of teaching styles.

In his book, *Teaching Martial Arts: the Way of the Master,* Dr. Sang Kim offers insight into maintaining student interest, which is presented in figure 2.1.

Teaching Children

"Kids love to compare and compete, and they especially love calling attention to each other's mistakes. I frequently have to remind them that I am the teacher and their job is to concentrate on their own improvement, without worrying about anyone else's... From the student's point of view, the problem is that the mind is quicker than the body—and the mouth is quicker than the mind." [13]

– Didi Goodman Sensei,
Chief Instructor,
Cuong Nhu Redwood dojo

Successful educational programs for children must accommodate their levels of physical and emotional growth. Martial arts can play an important role in helping children enhance their self-esteem, develop mental discipline, learn self-defense, and improve their physical conditioning. When younger children encounter a stimulating, enjoyable, and safe classroom environment, they will build solid foundations from which they can learn more advanced skills as they age.

In general, children have trouble remembering more than three things in a row. The older the child, the more complex instruction he or she will be able to retain. Regardless of age, however, children internalize instruction best when it is broken down into simple components. Complex techniques are best taught as a series of simple steps that, once mastered, can be reintegrated into a whole.

Dr. Sang Kim offers insight into the characteristics of various age groups and the appropriate teaching emphasis thereof. Although the following is not a direct quote, I draw heavily upon his work in offering this list:

Age 6–9, Characteristics and Teaching Emphasis

Characteristics:

- Active and energetic.
- Constrained by demands to conform to rules of etiquette and proper behavior.
- Aggressive with competitive tendencies becoming more prominent.
- Concerned about rules and organization.
- Confident of physical abilities yet tending to overestimate capabilities (accident rates peak at age nine).
- Eager to please teachers, admire teachers.
- Sensitive to criticism with difficulty in handling failure.
- Desirous of knowledge.

Teaching emphasis:

- Active participation (followed by rest periods as appropriate).
- Rough activities like punching or kicking a heavy bag to disperse aggression.
- Small group games (cooperative) with simple rules.
- Strict limits on acceptable behavior, especially during free-practice periods.
- Appoint helpers or leaders for each class to encourage leadership.
- Provide many opportunities for success in the classroom, praising success and avoiding negative criticism.
- Vary class activities from day to day, presenting skills in different and complementary ways.

Age 9–12, Characteristics and Teaching Emphasis

Characteristics:

- Physically, significant growth spurts in girls and some boys.
- Development of fine motor skills and better coordination.
- Begin the process of establishing an identity separate from parents.
- Desire for acceptance by peer group begins to replace adults as role model.
- Highly competitive with a strong desire for recognition.

Teaching emphasis:

- Begin teaching more complex skills and provide more detailed instruction.
- Utilize small group activities that encourage both cooperation and competition between groups.
- Create contests or games (e.g., arm wrestling, speed target punching or kicking, *kata* competition) that yield several winners; vary such activities

so that everyone has a chance to win.

- Design competitive activities with size/strength/gender differences in mind.
- Encourage responsible behavior and goal setting.
- Provide opportunities for self-directed learning.

Age 12–15, Characteristics and Teaching Emphasis

Characteristics:

- Growth spurts begin in boys.
- Girls excel in flexibility and balance while boys excel in strength, speed, and endurance.
- Peer group acceptance becomes a top priority.
- Great concern for physical appearance is expressed by both sexes.
- Self-image coalesces.
- Attention span lengthens significantly.
- Ability for sustained aerobic activity is developed.

Teaching emphasis:

- Begin teaching complex skills that require lengthy practice.
- Provide opportunities to teach others as skills develop.
- Encourage strengths and compensate for weaknesses.
- Encourage cooperative activities that demand problem solving and creativity for success.
- Give ample positive feedback and teach students how to improve themselves.
- Avoid negative criticism, especially of physical faults.

Games and Competitions

Contests, which can be very motivational for children, should be incorporated into the curricula so long as they serve legitimate educational purposes and everyone has an opportunity to win. There should never be a "loser" in any competition. My students particularly enjoy *kata* competitions where the winner earns the right to punch me in the stomach (it should be noted that the concept of using karate only for mental and physical conditioning or self-defense is continuously reinforced such that this reward is not misinterpreted as license for gratuitously hitting people outside the *dojo*). Since the senior students invariably do the best *kata* and I want to make opportunities available for everyone, I frequently use "*Sensei* Says" as well. This game is usually inserted at the very end of a class session to reinforce that day's lessons and wrap things up in a positive manner.

Played similarly to "*Simon Says*," students learn to pay careful attention to the instructor while practicing various *kihon* (basics or fundamental techniques). This game also helps students internalize karate terminology as I tend to call out techniques practiced earlier in the day using Japanese rather than English nomenclature (e.g., "*jodan tsuki*" rather than "head punch"). Initially, those who do not correctly perform the techniques (or do something other than what *sensei* says) earn five push-ups. Finally, as time runs out students who miss a move are simply out of the game until there is one overall winner.

While I frequently use individual contests, group competitions are also important. Another popular kid's game is called the "Gauntlet of Death," a group activity with no "winner" in and of itself. This game reinforces body alignment, movement, stance, guard, and striking techniques and is very popular. Although children (especially boys) love gory sounding activities, it is generally a good idea to get their parent's buy-in before using names like this. It is also important to stress that the opportunity to hit things during class does not give one license to propagate violence *outside* the *dojo*. Furthermore, such names should be presented with pacing, meter, and body language that reinforce your humorous intent (e.g., imitating the announcer at auto rally: "Thaaa Gauntlet.... Of Deeaath! … Deaath … Death!").

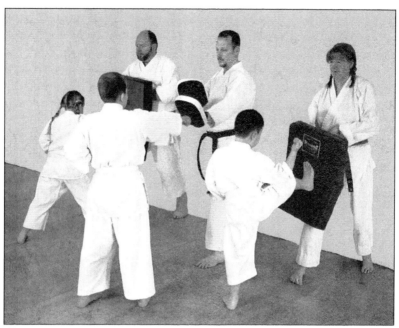

WHEN PLAYED AT THE END OF A TRAINING SESSION, THE "GAUNTLET OF DEATH" IS AN EXCEL-
LENT OPPORTUNITY TO BRING TOGETHER A VARIETY OF BASIC ELEMENTS THAT HAVE BEEN
PRACTICED INDEPENDENTLY THROUGHOUT A CLASS. I LIKE TO USE IT AS A REWARD FOR PAYING
ATTENTION AND TRAINING HARD DURING PREVIOUS PARTS OF THE SESSION.[D]

The game is played by having the instructors (and some of
the students when appropriate) stand in a long line holding
various pads or shields while students participating in the
gauntlet run from person to person punching or kicking each
target. (If students are needed to form the gauntlet, be sure
that those students also have the opportunity to run through
it as well). Sometimes, we incorporate a heavy bag or two as
part of the line. Students are typically given specific
techniques to practice along the gauntlet, though at the end of
the session they are usually given free reign to practice whatever they like. When students drop their guard or turn their
backs on an instructor as they run past, they are struck (light-
ly) with the pad.

Board breaking is another competition enjoyed by students. Children love to break boards, and I have found that it
significantly reinforces their self-esteem. To keep the cost

down, we use re-breakable boards made out of plastic. The degree of difficulty in "breaking" these devices can be adjusted by changing the center bar that holds the two halves together. If the person holding the board torques it a bit, almost any age child can break it with their strike, even if they don't follow-through properly. For safety reasons, we have newer or younger students attack the board with a palm-heel strike (*shotei uchi*) so that their hands will not be seriously hurt if they do not punch all the way through. As children advance in rank and experience we can crank-up the degree of difficulty so that only proper technique and good follow-through will break the board.

I actually use a larger variety of games/competitions than the few examples listed here. While the *dojo* is not a place to entertain children, lessons must be orchestrated in a manner that engages their full attention throughout each session. Where contests serve a legitimate educational purpose, I integrate them to reinforce my lesson plans.

Teaching Adults

"Many new students can envision wearing a black belt and feeling the pride and confidence such an accomplishment brings. Soon after students begin instruction, they are hit with the reality that most beginning training borders on the mundane. Most "traditional" martial arts schools teach beginning students in the same manner: there is a steady dose of form, basic mechanical technique, and repetitive kicking and punching drills. The result is that the initial excitement wears thin, and the grand vision of mastery is sometimes lost." [14]

– *Tracy Tucker Sensei*

While teaching children can be a lot like filling empty vessels with facts and ideas, teaching experienced adults is much more complex. Concepts can no longer simply be poured in;

they must be fitted into what is already there. As continuous learners who generally know the modalities by which they learn best (even if they cannot articulate them well), adults gravitate toward instructors whose training methods reach them effectively.

Adults become ready to learn when they experience the need to know. Consequently, they expect the learning to be meaningful and directly applicable to their goals. Curricula should present opportunities to apply new skills in meaningful ways with appropriate feedback from fellow learners and instructors.

Adult beginners frequently seek out martial arts to get back into shape, stay in shape, learn self-defense, or find relief from the stresses of work or family life. They are often self-conscious and incessantly aware of their level of ability and speed of learning. As a result, the learning environment should stress personal development, perseverance, and positive feedback. For classes focused upon self-defense techniques, ethical and legal components must be emphasized as well.

Proper Warm-Up

While adults also have characteristics inherent to their age, differences important for martial arts instruction primarily relate to learning style and physical ability. Unlike younger children, it is especially important to provide adequate warm-up time prior to vigorous physical activity to minimize the possibility of muscle, tendon, or joint injury during training. Adequate cool down should also be emphasized.

This warm-up may be incorporated into the course curricula and done as a group. In the group setting, certain students may perform better and more correctly than they would on their own. When initially learning *daruma* (exercise) techniques, it is important that students receive hands-on tutelage to ensure that they are doing them properly and will not inadvertently injure themselves. Once they know how to perform warm-ups correctly, adult students may be expected to complete their exercises individually prior to the beginning of class. This alternative approach leaves more class time available that can be devoted to teaching martial technique. Cool-down stretching is almost always performed solo after class.

Mastering the Basics

While basic drills are the foundation of martial arts technique, sufficient variety must be inserted into class curricula to maintain student interest. It is useful to describe the practice of these basics as an ascending spiral. Each time a student repeats the drill, he or she will incorporate a higher level of understanding which, in essence, allows the student to approach the technique in a whole new way. Theoretically, a technique may be practiced 100 times or 100 techniques may be practiced only once, as each is different and more evolved than the one that came before. While it is essential to practice the basics on a regular basis, *kihon* should not be the sole agenda of any class session.

As advanced students coalesce their understanding of martial techniques, they begin to appreciate how little they have truly mastered. Basic punches, kicks, and footwork take on a whole new meaning when students integrate their bodies and begin to utilize internal energy rather than brute muscle force. The subtlety and nuance necessary to punch or kick "properly" can only be developed through disciplined, repetitive practice. Once they reach a certain level of understanding, students will generally begin to practice the basics on their own, making time for repetitions not covered in formal class sessions.

Summary

World-class educators account for differences in student personalities and react accordingly to facilitate communication. The MBTI tool helps educators understand the role of individual differences in personality type and how to accommodate all of them in instruction. It is particularly helpful to understand an individual's preference toward Extroversion or Introversion and his or her inclination toward Sensing or Intuition, two of eight dichotomous dimensions identified by the MBTI tool. This helps instructors understand the degree to which students feel comfortable asking questions and the extent to which they need to know how and/or why something works before attempting it. Active listening is another important skill for deciphering student personality types and understanding their learning predilections.

Personality differences play a significant role in effectively motivating *budoka* as well. To be most effective, motivational techniques must be adapted to the individual. In general, however, one can motivate beginners by teaching a variety of simple skills in a straightforward manner while providing regular, positive reinforcement. For intermediate students, instructors should begin to introduce the history and philosophy of the art form and individualize training methods to the extent practicable. For advanced students, instructors should broaden knowledge through training and provide opportunities for these students to teach other students. Remember that personality differences aside, adults tend to be more intrinsically motivated, requiring less handholding than children in educational situations.

Although the teaching emphasis for children will vary by age group, games and competitions can fortify the curricula so long as they serve a legitimate educational purpose and everyone has an opportunity to win. Recall that teaching children is a lot like filling empty vessels with facts and ideas, whereas teaching experienced adults is more complex. For adults concepts must be meaningful and directly applicable to their goals It must also be fitted into what is already there. Curricula should present opportunities to apply new skills in a meaningful way with appropriate feedback from fellow learners and instructors.

CHAPTER 3

Application of the Six Teaching Styles to ✳ Martial Arts ✳

"You cannot teach a man anything. You can only help him discover it within himself." [15]

– Galileo

Understanding learning-style differences is only one component of exemplary teaching. It does not matter what you know or how much you know if you cannot communicate it effectively. Educators have a variety of teaching styles available with which they can effectively convey their knowledge. Different styles are appropriate for different applications. Competent instructors will match appropriate teaching styles to the situations for which those styles are best suited. The six main teaching styles are:

- Modeling
- Lecturing
- Cooperative performance
- Independent performance
- Knowledge capture
- Role reversal

The following section briefly describes each teaching style, its appropriate application, and how to apply it when teaching martial arts. The key is flexibility to adopt the style best suited to the type of information the instructor is trying to convey.

---

(1) Modeling

"The first thing I learned from Higa was how to walk in Sanchin Dachi (basic "hourglass" stance). The exercise was monotonous and boring but repeated numerous times until Sensei approved." [16]

– Seikichi Toguchi Sensei

In modeling, the instructor applies his or her expertise to a current task while the student observes the instructor's actions. The student learns by observation and should record as much of the instructor's performance as possible so that it can become a model of how the student should perform the task.

When to Model

Modeling may be a good method to initiate a new teaching relationship, as the instructor simply does what he or she does best and the student learns by observing. It can be particularly useful when an instructor is having difficulty verbally describing his or her knowledge but does not have difficulty performing it, when language barriers inhibit communication, when the student needs to acquire information that emphasizes the sequential and simultaneous organization of a task's details, or when the student needs to follow a series of typically nonverbal, non-documented procedures in order to complete a task.

Application of Modeling to Martial Arts

Traditionally, instruction of karate, aikido, kung fu, judo, and related Asian martial arts relies heavily on modeling relationships. Students observe and attempt to imitate their *sensei's* techniques, transcending potential language barriers and other inhibiters of communication. This is a particularly powerful method of introducing students to the gross physical patterns of *kata, bunkai, kiso kumite, kihon,* and other applications (e.g., strikes, blocks, stances, and movement).

Once the basics are understood, however, other teaching methods will generally be required to communicate the subtlety, depth, and nuance of a technique (e.g., proper breathing, stance dynamics, hidden strikes within blocks, hidden blocks within strikes, pressure point/nerve techniques; and advanced moving, shifting, seeking, or blending techniques).

---
(2) Lecturing

"Beginning in 1952, Miyagi's health severely declined. When he taught us, he always sat in a chair and orally instructed us one at a time." [17]

– Seikichi Toguchi Sensei

In lecturing, the instructor verbally and visually presents information in a direct instructional format to the student. Handouts, books, articles, web sites, and videotapes are additional resources that the instructor can assign.

When to Lecture

Complete descriptions of expertise are required for lecturing. Consequently, lecturing is appropriate when the instructor's knowledge can be verbally and visually presented in an organized and comprehensive manner. Lecturing is particularly useful when the student does not have a strong foundation of a concept and needs to acquire this knowledge (e.g., facts, concepts, relationships among concepts, and declarative information). This technique is especially powerful when a student is initially learning new material and must understand a general framework within which to integrate the details.

Application of Lecturing to Martial Arts

Lecturing is particularly useful when describing the history or strategic approach of a martial art or communicating similar conceptual frameworks. For example, in *Goju Ryu* the strategy is to stay close to an opponent, keep that opponent off balance, and use physiological incapacitation to defeat the opponent. When a practitioner can incapacitate his or her opponent's vision, breathing, or movement, the practitioner is in an excellent position to defeat that enemy. Any two out of three will pretty much guarantee success. Such (strategic) concepts cannot be understood intuitively nor can they be readily interpolated from watching other people demonstrate individual martial techniques (tactics).

Another example of an appropriate subject to teach via lecturing is the concept of *kaisai no genri*, the work of finding hidden techniques within *kata* (see "Teaching Bunkai"). While *kata* is composed of many apparent movements of fighting techniques, or *hyomengi*, many of these movements are stylized with the actual application hidden. The theory of *kaisai* provides karate practitioners a basis from which to identify and understand these hidden techniques. *Bunkai*, or application of such technique, would generally be communicated through cooperative performance and/or independent study.

---
(3) Cooperative Performance

"I see now that with the approach of his death, he (Miyagi) felt the time was right to impart his secret theories of karate to me. These theories included Kaisai no Genri (the theory of karate kata), how to create Hookiyu (unified) kata, and the concept of creating and developing a teaching system for karate." [18]

– *Seikichi Toguchi Sensei*

In cooperative performance, the instructor and student work side by side on a task, engaging in a continuous discussion on how to do something. The student can learn basic facts and concepts and can obtain guided practice on how to perform a task. The style and balance of the continuous discussions can be varied to meet particular goals of the instructor and student. Sometimes the instructor should initiate the performance, with the student asking questions and other times the student should initiate the performance, with the instructor providing feedback and commentary.

When to Cooperatively Perform

For cooperative performance to be effective, the student should already have some basic competencies in performing the task. Cooperation works best in situations where the student needs to learn situation-specific information that only becomes available while one is performing a task, needs to learn the ways that the instructor makes some of the subtle judgments required by a task, or needs to learn to identify the factors that influence the instructor's choice of a particular tactic in a particular situation. Another situation that calls for cooperative learning is when the student needs to learn *why* the instructor is thinking about a problem in a specific manner.

Application of Cooperative Performance to Martial Arts

Cooperative performance can be a powerful tool to help students understand how to apply martial tactics, such as *bunkai,* within the framework of an art's strategy. When working various *kumite* (sparring) drills such as line sparring or *randori* (free sparring), it is often useful to discuss what works, what does not work, and why that is the case in conjunction with application of the technique(s). This can help students develop a better understanding of which approaches are most effective for someone of their size, conditioning, skill level, and body type.

As they build a repertoire of techniques to draw from, advanced students will need to develop an understanding of how and when to combine or modify movements as they face varying tactical environments and prepare for real-life self-defense situations. While this could certainly be accomplished through trial and error during *kumite* or *randori,* cooperative performance will add significant velocity to the learning process. It is generally less painful that way too.

(4) Independent Performance

"Solo training clearly offers a wide range of benefits to martial artists. Whereas class sessions are designed to meet the needs of a group, solo practice is designed for the individual, around his schedule... The two approaches are meant to supplement each other in order to produce a more well-rounded practitioner." [19]

– Jimmie Nixdorf Sensei

Here, the instructor assigns a specific task for the student to complete and the instructor evaluates the student's end performance, providing feedback as necessary. Independent performance is most appropriate when the student needs to learn to make his or her own judgment in completing a known task or goal.

When to Independently Perform:

For complex tasks, the student should have gained at least at an intermediate level of expertise and should have developed some skills and procedural knowledge. Independent performance facilitates development of a student's confidence in his or her own judgment and helps the student to trust his or her own skills. It can help a student learn to evaluate his or her own performance and thinking abilities, promoting meta-cognitive skill development. The student can independently assess the successfulness a strategy against a desired task, outcome, or goal.

Application of Independent Performance to Martial Arts

Independent performance is an excellent opportunity for more advanced students to internalize and further develop previous learning. Students should be taught to practice their art form a little bit each day. As they struggle to remember movements of a *kata* or define applications for a technique, students can take real ownership of the knowledge they discover and learn confidence from their achievements. No matter how many times a strategy, technique, or application is explained by an instructor, there is nothing like experiencing the concept for one's self to truly understand and internalize it.

Many new students become leery of performing independently prior to understanding techniques at an intermediate or higher level. The most common fear is that of "learning it wrong" as most assume that once something has been learned incorrectly it becomes difficult, if not impossible, to correct. To help students overcome this concern and facilitate their abilities to progress more quickly, I occasionally assign homework to individual students. It might be something as simple as watching television for ten minutes while standing in a particular stance, or hitting a punching bag a certain number of times using a particular technique. This homework is always based on something they know well enough to practice properly, but for which additional improvement is still necessary. Once a pattern of independent training has been established, most students incorporate it into their daily habits.

Another important aspect of independent performance in martial arts is training under a variety of conditions beyond the familiar environment of the *dojo* floor. As a yellow belt I went on vacation to the Philippines for month. Not wanting to forget what I had recently learned in class and wanting to help myself recover from the nineteen-hour plane ride, I went outside to practice my *kata*. As it was 90 degrees and 90 percent humidity outside, I chose to wear shorts and sandals.

It was a bit of a shock to discover that training with shoes outdoors, on an uneven surface under the blazing sun is nothing like practicing with bare feet on a smooth wooden floor wearing a traditional *gi* during winter time in Seattle. While that should have been obvious, I simply had not considered the differences before experiencing them.

Years later I still try to regularly practice on a variety of indoor and outdoor surfaces, wearing an assortment of footgear and clothing, so that if I ever need to utilize my skills in a defensive manner, I will not be caught off guard by the environmental conditions under which I am attacked. A certain degree of prudence is required when practicing martial arts in a public venue, however, so as to not inadvertently provoke a real fight.

In the *dojo*, it is traditional to start every *kata* facing *shomen* (front). I have found that it is prudent to occasionally begin a *kata* facing some other direction (or even to practice with one's eyes closed) to acclimate to other perspectives. The first time I tried this it was quite a challenge.

---

(5) Knowledge Capture

> *"...After the third forward step and punch with left hand, pull the left hand back past your nipple and then bring it under the right elbow (your elbow is on top of the left wrist). At the same time you place your right foot diagonally in front of the left foot in order to be able to stand in correct Sanchin Dachi after turning (at this foot position the legs are crossed). Then quickly turn on the ball of the foot as if you are pressing both feet into the ground. After completing the turn, execute a right-hand punch..."* [20]

> – *Chojun Miyagi Sensei*
> *from his writing "Goju-Ryu Kenpo,"*
> *a treatise on Sanchin kata written in 1932*

With knowledge capture, the translation from a mental mode to physical medium stimulates a coalescence of understanding and facilitates a logical organization of the knowledge documented. The student designs instructional materials that represent his or her expertise, the important and subtle environmental cues used to perform and mediate skill, feedback methods that are monitored to ensure the success of performance and thinking processes, and/or the general knowledge and skills that the student would use to cope with novel problems. Typically, this is more official than mere note-taking yet not always as formal as developing a proper seminar or thesis.

When to Capture Knowledge and Expertise

Knowledge capture is most appropriate when the student has advanced knowledge and skills, performs consistently and well, yet needs to improve conceptualization and organized understanding of the expertise. Through knowledge capture, the student learns to gather the general principles that organize all the component tasks learned and to communicate that information to others in an effective manner. Additionally, when the student has to solve many novel problems, he or she needs to learn a set of general strategies to approach and successfully solve new problems.

Application of Knowledge Capture to Martial Arts

As with *Goju Ryu* karate, many martial art forms require advanced students to complete a thesis project concurrent with testing for *dan* (black belt) rank. This is an excellent opportunity for these individuals to advance the knowledge base of their organizations while clarifying and adding depth to their own understanding of their chosen martial arts. As students progress through the lower ranks, it is very useful for them to document what they have learned in journals or notebooks. The mere process of writing things down facilitates internalization and understanding of the knowledge that is written. The ultimate progression of knowledge capture is the publication of books and/or articles about one's art.

Over the years I have developed an extensive collection of notes about the martial forms I have practiced. Since I type much faster than I can write by hand, most of them are available electronically so that I can make copies for students who ask. Not only has this helped codify my own knowledge, but I have also found that I can easily share essential materials with members of my class who want them.

---
(6) Role Reversal
---

*"So, following his principles, I created Gekiha
Dai Ichi and Gekiha Dai Ni kata. I showed them to*

my teacher Higa and my Sempai Mr. Meitoku Yagi. They both approved and felt it was what Miyagi Sensei was striving for." [21]

– *Seikichi Toguchi Sensei*

For each of the previous five instructional interactions, the student and instructor can exchange roles. For example, the student might model, performing an entire task while the instructor observes. In this manner, the instructor can determine how well a student has developed his or her procedural knowledge and how well the student has learned to react to situational cues. The student may lecture while the instructor evaluates how well the student understands the knowledge domain. Similarly, an instructor may perform independently while the student evaluates how the instructor performed a task and how successfully he or she completed it.

When to use Role Reversal

Many instructors find role reversal a very effective and fun process for verifying students' knowledge and skills. Role reversal is effective in a variety of situations and, in most cases, may be used with all but the most junior of students. Additionally, an instructor may wish to capture and share his or her own knowledge about the role reversal. This step might be important where students do not have the time to develop the level of expertise necessary to understand or document abstract principles, particularly when a handbook, notes, procedures, or written instructions would facilitate the learning process.

Application of Role Reversal to Martial Arts

The most common use of role reversal in martial arts is when the instructor asks individual students to lead portions of a class (e.g., *daruma*, *kata*, *kiso kumite*, or *kata bunkai*). Additionally, senior students are usually asked to practice with junior students, helping them advance their skills. By teaching others, students internalize the material and develop a deeper understanding of the techniques they instruct. They also help

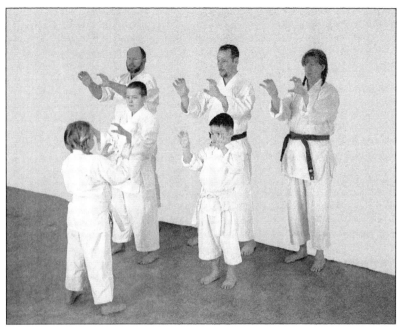

BY TEACHING OTHERS, STUDENTS INTERNALIZE THE MATERIAL AND DEVELOP A DEEPER UNDER-
STANDING OF THE TECHNIQUES THEY DEMONSTRATE. HERE, A JUNIOR STUDENT LEADS THE
CLASS THROUGH *DARUMA*. THE GRIPPING EXERCISE SHE IS DIRECTING STRENGTHENS PRACTI-
TIONER'S HANDS AND FOREARMS. [E]

their instructor ensure a productive classroom environment by
accommodating a variety skill levels simultaneously, making
efficient use of class time, and optimizing personal attention
that the instructor has with each student. Role reversal can be
used for both children's and adult's classes.

Summary

Teachers have a variety of styles available with which they
can effectively communicate their knowledge. Like tools in a
workshop, different teaching styles are appropriate for different applications. The six main teaching styles—modeling, lecturing, cooperative performance, independent performance,
knowledge capture, and role reversal—are directly applicable
to the instruction of martial arts. Proficient instructors will
match each approach to the situation(s) for which it is best
suited.

For example, traditional instruction in Asian martial arts relies heavily upon modeling relationships where students observe and attempt to imitate their *sensei's* techniques, transcending potential language barriers and other inhibiters of communication. While this is a particularly powerful method of introducing students to the gross physical movements of an art form, lecturing is required to communicate essential strategic frameworks as well as important nuances of individual tactics or techniques (e.g., stance dynamics, internal power, *sanchin* breathing, or pressure point/nerve manipulation).

Cooperative and independent performance set in motion a trial and error process through which students develop a better understanding of which techniques are most effective for their unique physical attributes and abilities. Under knowledge capture, the mere process of writing down information facilitates internalization and understanding of the knowledge. By teaching others via role reversal, students internalize the materials taught and develop even deeper understanding.

CHAPTER 4

Fostering a Positive
✳ Learning Environment ✳

*"It takes two to speak the truth—one to speak
and another to hear."* [22]

– Henry David Thoreau

The general mindset and biases of the people with whom educators plan to share information will color what they can hear and how they hear it. These are both intellectual as well as emotional. The influences on how people will interpret what an instructor presents include:

- Their previous experience with and attitude about the subject matter.
- What is urgent and important to them at the time of instruction.
- The mental models through which they make sense of the world.
- Any previous experience they might have had (or may have heard about) with the instructor.
- Any outside issues that may distract their attention.
- Semantics, language, and terminology.

In the summer of 1996 I was teaching a Microsoft Excel (a popular spreadsheet application) class at Renton Technical College. During this class, I received a very important, unexpected lesson about mental models, individual bias, and student perception.

First, some important background to set the stage: due to a remodeling project that was running a bit behind schedule, the school's air conditioning was not working particularly well. The temperature had reached about 85 degrees during the day (considerably warmer than normal for that time of the year), with heat lingering well into the evening. Consequently I left the classroom doors and windows open to increase airflow and help the students to be comfortable enough to pay attention despite the unusually warm weather.

After taking care of the required *"administrivia"* at the beginning of each new class session, I had developed a routine of having the students introduce themselves, and briefly discuss their backgrounds, experience, and expectations for the course in order that I might tailor the materials to best meet their collective needs and skill level. Normally when a student comes in late, I would become aware of his or her presence either by seeing them pass-through the door or by hearing it open or close. On that particular night, however, a student slipped into the room while I had my back to the door writing on the whiteboard. Not hearing her come in, I was unaware or her tardy arrival. I did not really notice at the time, but it is important to point out that the late student was a person of Asian-American descent.

Once we had completed the introductions, I asked if I had missed anyone, not because I expected that I had, but just be sure that I had not left anyone out (another habit born from adverse experience). Naturally the student who had come in late raised her hand. Somewhat surprised, I nevertheless asked her to tell the class her name, what she did when not taking classes at the college, her computer experience, her spreadsheet experience, and her expectations for the course.

Once she was finished introducing herself, I asked everyone to turn to page three of their handbook so that we could begin. A minute or two later she stopped me, saying that she did not have the class materials I was referring to. Again, I was slightly taken aback, as I still had not realized that she had come in late. I was certain that everyone already had a copy since I had previously checked before putting the extras back into the file cabinet. Nevertheless, I double-checked to make sure that no one else was missing a copy then retrieved one from the office for her before proceeding to move on through the course material that I had intended to present.

Halfway through that day's session we had a ten-minute break during which someone pointed out to me that the student in question had arrived late. He had clearly noted the puzzled look on my face when the tardy student told me that she did not have a handout and had decided to tell me what had happened. At the time I thought the whole incident was kind of funny, but did not think it would have any significance. In that light, I found it somewhat unusual that the previously tardy student did not return from the break, but again did not think that it was any big deal. After all, people would occasionally drop out of the first class after I reviewed the syllabus because they realized that the material would be too difficult, too easy, or otherwise would not fit their needs. I gave the incident no further thought. Boy was I ever wrong!

That first class was on a Monday. Thursday morning I received a call from the Associate Dean for whom I worked informing me that she had received a ten-page (single-space, ten point font) letter from a disgruntled *"former"* student who had attended the first session of my Excel class. This student accused me, among other things, of belittling her, making her share personal information in front of the entire class, and refusing to provide her with necessary classroom materials. She further claimed I was a misogynist, a racist, and a bigot.

Obviously I was shocked, as would be anyone who knew me. Fortunately I had six years experience and a history of outstanding performance reviews at the college. I was well known to my employer as an honorable, unbiased person who respected diversity and treated students fairly. Furthermore, I was also (and still am) married to an Asian American.

To make a long story much, much shorter, everyone lived happily ever after except for the lawyers who ended up having nothing to do. Had my background or tenure been any different, however, it may not have turned out that way.

Some people go through life carrying a giant chip on their shoulder. Clearly this woman believed that she had been discriminated against or otherwise horribly wronged in the past. Consequently, she approached new situations with a very different mindset than most people would expect. While I still may not really understand it to this day, her perspective was certainly legitimate for her at that time.

What is important to take away from this story is that what an instructor communicates may be materially divergent from what his or her students receive and understand. While educators cannot control the biases and perceptions of their students, they certainly can take responsibility for communicating as clearly as they know how. More importantly, they must take responsibility for their own attitudes regarding this communication. If the student does not understand, it is almost always the teacher's fault. Keeping this in mind will make for much stronger communicators, as demonstrated by the next vignette.

Attitude

"… So as you can see, there is more than one right way to do almost everything in Excel. There is also more than one right way to explain how to do almost everything. I will do my best to make sure that everyone is on the same page, using explanations I have found effective in the past. Nevertheless, if an explanation doesn't work for you, that's OK. Just let me know that you're lost and I'll try it a different way until you are found. You are paying a lot of money to be here and it is my job to give you your money's worth. In other words, if you don't get it, it's my fault…

"That's extremely important, so I'll say it again: If you don't get it, it's my fault! But, if you are lost and you don't ask a question then it's your fault. Fair enough?" [23]

– Lawrence Kane
Introduction to MS Excel
Renton Technical College

When I first began teaching software courses in 1990, I was very well prepared. I had previous substitute teaching experience, had taken the required education courses, and had successfully passed all the State certification requirements to teach. An expert in my subject area, I had spent months developing the course curricula, testing the class materials, and *"bullet-proofing"* my approach. As a former consultant and Educational Vice President of Toastmasters International, I had already given countless presentations to a variety of audiences and was confident of my ability to perform in a classroom environment. I was also very excited about the opportunity to teach part-time, as the pay was nearly three times the salary of my full-time job at the time, and I really needed the extra income.

I taught two 30-hour classes per academic quarter, each with two 3-hour sessions per week. The first three quarters went reasonably well. Grading was competency based and generally pass/fail, though letter grades were available for individuals who needed them (e.g., tuition reimbursement). During that time period, roughly 70% of my students passed my course with 20% dropping out early and 10% receiving failing grades. That seemed pretty good at the time.

Once students completed the final examination on the last session of each class, they had an opportunity to complete a confidential evaluation form that was later reviewed by the Associate Dean of the Business Technology Department at the school. My evaluations over those first three academic quarters were about average when compared to my peer instructors in the department. Perhaps not outstanding scores, but pretty good nevertheless.

I overcame some interesting challenges during at this time as well including one Russian gentleman who spoke no English, not one word, yet nevertheless successfully passed the course. Fortunately, he was Jewish and spoke a little Yiddish, a language comprised primarily of German and Hebrew. As he struggled to speak Yiddish, I replied in broken German, utilizing what little I remembered from high school. It was terribly comical, but it worked. And, to a large degree, it entertained the other students rather than annoying them.

I also graduated two additional non-English speakers who brought translators to class along with a quadriplegic who managed to type using a special pen he held in his mouth. If I could overcome that, I could do anything! I was "Superteacher", or so I thought... About halfway through the fourth quarter, everything changed.

To truly appreciate what happened, it is important to understand the demographics of my class and the lens through which I viewed them. My students fell into three major categories—roughly one third were recent high school graduates looking to brush up on job skills as they entered the workplace. One third of my students were parents of high school aged children looking to return to the workplace after taking time off to raise their kids. The remaining third were (primarily) clerical and professional employees trying to enhance their job skills, either to take advantage of promotional opportunities or to perform adequately in their current position.

While the public education system had not yet reached its current state of disarray, very few high school students at that time graduated with any significant degree of computer literacy. This third of the class certainly were not stupid, but they were generally undereducated, minimally motivated, immature, and had a propensity to drift off subject to inconsequential things that disrupted the class. On top of that, many were young, single parents living on welfare, who had significant challenges with punctuality if not attendance. Because I had to sign a special form affirming their presence in class each week, I knew which students were receiving state assistance and I suspect this did not positively influence my perception of them.

The second third of the class tended to be terrified of all things computer, truly believing they could launch a nuclear holocaust from their PC (ala the movie *War Games*) or otherwise inflict terrible disasters upon themselves or others. It may be hard to believe today, but back in 1990 most of these students began the class having never used or seen a computer, frequently believing that a mouse was furry rodent and that a keyboard belonged on a typewriter. These people were certainly not obtuse in any way, but I had a very low tolerance for what

I considered *"stupidity"* at that time of my life and I probably treated them as if they were in fact stupid, much to my later regret.

The last third of the student population were the highly motivated individuals upon whom I focused most of my time and energy. These folks were the most similar to me in professionalism, perspective, and perseverance. They tended to be eager, punctual, and hardworking. Consequently I held a natural affinity toward them.

One night after class, about midway through the session, I discovered one of my students sitting on the parking lot curb, head in hands, crying. She was a member of the *"third"* group. I assumed that she was a professional of some sort as she wore a suit to class every day. At first I thought that she had been injured in some way, but that turned-out not to be the case. When I asked her what was wrong, she told me that her job was in jeopardy because she was not learning the material well enough.

It turns out that she worked for a local insurance company as a secretary. They had recently purchased several personal computers to replace the mainframe terminals they had previously used to complete their work. They wanted everyone to learn how to use personal productivity software such as WordPerfect® (a word processing program) and Lotus 1-2-3® (spreadsheet software) that came with the new machines (this was back before Microsoft dominated the industry). Because her boss was unwilling to expend any money to train employees, this student had taken it upon herself to attend classes at night and then teach her coworkers what she had learned the next morning.

Unfortunately, her boss had come to expect that she would be able to teach him whatever he could not figure out on his own and was asking questions about material that she did not fully understand or had not been introduced to yet. Worse still, he had already threatened to fire her if she could not solve his problems in a timely manner. In fact, now that they had these *"powerful new computers,"* he told her that he was not sure why it was necessary to keep a secretary at all. If she could not change her job, she felt that she would undoubtedly lose it.

In answer to the obvious, *"So why don't you just quit and find a new job?"* question, she told me that she had been working there long enough that she made far more than she could expect to receive at other companies. Since her husband had decided to return to school full-time after being laid off, she said that she could not cover her family's bills with anything less, at least not until he graduated.

Clearly I felt bad for her situation, but what really shocked me was that I had thought she was doing quite well in the class. She worked steadily, invariably finished her projects correctly and on-time, and asked few questions. She may have needed more in-depth understanding than others in the class, but I really thought she was doing fine. Unfortunately I discovered that, in most cases, she was able to follow step-by-step directions but did not truly understanding what she was doing and why it worked.

At that moment I had a true epiphany. If this hardworking, well-dressed, obviously intelligent individual did not truly understand my lessons, how many others had I lost as well? This really bothered me, not only because I felt badly for my student, but also because it made me question how effectively I had really been communicating. I thought that I had accounted for every learning style preference and most any contingency in my lesson plans, yet somehow it was not enough. What it all boiled down to, I came to realize, was not technique. It was attitude.

Until that point I had believed that there truly were "stupid" questions. Since I had learned the topics quite easily and had been exercising such perfect technique in communicating them, only a true "idiot" could not grasp the concepts as easily as I.

Obviously I had been the one acting "stupidly" and had finally come to realize it. My students were paying big money to learn how to use the software. I was responsible for giving them their money's worth. Not only that, but I owed them patience, effective listening, and clear communication. In other words, if they didn't get it, it was MY fault, not theirs.

I came to understand that since there was more than one "right" way to do everything in the software (e.g., the formula 'C1+C2+C3 in a Lotus 1-2-3 spreadsheet works identically to the formula @sum(C1:C3), which equates to =sum(C1:C3) in Excel®), there must be more than one "right" way to explain how to do it. I knew that I was smart enough to figure out an alternate way to describe whatever a student might not understand. I was able to boil my epiphany down to a simple phrase, which is quoted at the beginning of this section, "If you don't get it, it's my fault."

Through my conversation with one distraught student I had come to internalize and believe this simple phrase. Later on, I started using that expression at the beginning of each new class session and frequently throughout the quarter. Eventually I also added the caveat, "But if you don't ask the question, then it's your fault," as I still have not mastered the art of reading minds.

Regardless of the phraseology, the point remains the same: educators are responsible for making sure that their students have every opportunity to understand the information they have enrolled to learn. We cannot bemoan, belittle, become irritated about, or ignore their legitimate needs to learn. We must exercise patience until we find effective way of communicating to each student directly. They do, after all, pay our salaries.

After that attitude correction on my part, my student's grades dramatically improved. Dropout rates consistently fell to below 8 percent, frequently reaching zero. Between 1991 and 1998, when I retired from teaching, I only had to fail three students who could not successfully learn the materials. My evaluations rapidly rose toward the highest ratings of anyone in the Business Technology Department, among both full-time and part-time instructors, and stayed there consistently. More importantly perhaps, I received student accolades, thank-you notes, and letters commending me for communicating effectively, demonstrating patience, and fostering a positive learning environment.

This was the same course, taught by the same instructor,

using the same materials and the same instructional techniques, with the same preparation, yet with dramatically different results. It really is all in the attitude.

Etiquette

"If the spirit of humility, an intrinsic element of Bushido, is removed from the teaching of classical martial studies, the lack of this important virtue makes such studies mere systems of violence." [24]

– Dr. Inazo Nitobe

Reishiki comes from two Japanese words. The first is *rei*, which is defined as: bow, salutation, salute, courtesy, propriety, thanks, and appreciation. The second part of the term is *shiki*, which is defined as a ceremony, rite, or function. Combined, the term *reishiki* can translate as etiquette or manners.

Etiquette is an integral part of *budo*, for without it we would be practicing nothing more than base violence. Watching senior student's behavior during training and in their general actions and interactions in the *dojo* is a great way to learn *reishiki*, (provided that the senior students themselves have also been observant over the years, of course). The more training a person receives the calmer, more dignified, and humble that *karateka* (karate practitioner) should become. Students who practice etiquette ultimately make themselves better people as well as better martial artists.

Etiquette is demonstrated when students show respect for the following:

- Their *dojo*
- Their instructor(s)
- Their fellow students
- Themselves

Respect for the Dojo

It is essential that students respect the *dojo* where they train, as well as *dojos* they might visit for seminars, tournaments, or other activities. The behaviors of students reflect on their instructors as much as it does upon themselves. One should bow upon entering and leaving a *dojo*. Shoes and mundane clothing should be folded and left neatly by the door. Everyone should help keep the *dojo* neat and clean, putting away equipment at the end of each class session, when they are done using it, or at other appropriate times. Food and drinks should not be taken onto the *dojo* floor. Practitioners should face away from the *shomen* (front of the *dojo*) or senior students/teachers when adjusting their *gi's* (uniforms). And, of course, no one should ever swear or use inappropriate language in class.

Respect for One's Instructors

It is also essential that students respect their instructor(s), both the head instructor and any visiting *yudansha* (black belts) or assistant instructors. Students should be taught to bow before and after receiving instruction and to pay attention and be polite during class. Practitioners should try to follow along even when they do not understand exactly what to do; in other words, "if in doubt, fake it." Newer students can determine when and how it is appropriate to ask questions by emulating senior students.

Students should always strive to arrive at class on time. If someone arrives after the class has already started, he or she should quietly warm up and wait for the instructor's invitation to bow in and join the class.

Since the instructors are often quite busy, it is always appreciated when students volunteer to help set-up and tear down the room and do other administrative tasks (e.g., taking role) as needed. Instructors, in turn, should never abuse their position by taking advantage of student volunteers in an unethical or inappropriate manner (e.g., coercing someone into remodeling the *dojo* at no recompense).

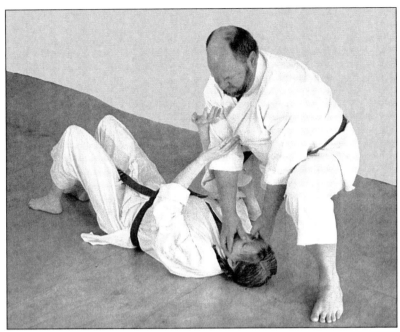

THERE ARE NO WEIGHT CLASS, SOCIAL CLASS, GENDER, AGE OR OTHER ARTIFICIAL RESTRIC-
TIONS IN A REAL FIGHT. CONSEQUENTLY, WE MUST ALL TRAIN TOGETHER AS *BUDOKA*. AS SUCH,
WE MUTUALLY DEMONSTRATE RESPECT, TRUST, AND COOPERATION IN LEARNING DANGEROUS
AND/OR DEADLY TECHNIQUES. THE *DOJO* AFFORDS US A SECURE ENVIRONMENT WHERE WE CAN
"THUMP" ON EACH OTHER WHILE PROTECTING OURSELVES, AND OUR TRAINING PARTNERS,
FROM SERIOUS INJURIES.[F]

Respect for Fellow Students

Martial arts practitioners should always be polite and show
respect their fellow students. They should be taught that it is
always appropriate to help those who know less than they do
and to learn from those who know more. In the *dojo*, we are
all *karateka*, so it is important to treat both males and females
in the same manner. All students should bow before and after
practicing together.

Students should be taught to line up according to rank at
the beginning and end of class, showing respect to elders and
deference to those of higher rank. In this manner, newer students will always know where to look and who to imitate if
they become lost or confused. When lined-up formally, students should be taught to go around the rows, rather than
walking between them if they are asked to approach the

shomen. If a student arrives late for class or forgets to bring their *obi* (belt), he or she should line up in the back—both at the beginning and end of class.

Respect for Oneself

Most importantly, practitioners must respect themselves. *Karateka* must understand that they need to ensure a proper balance and harmony between home life, work life, and martial arts practice. They should be sure that their *gi's* are clean and neat. Everyone must know his or her physical condition and practice accordingly, thoroughly warming up prior to training in order to avoid injury, and properly cooling-down after. Students should work hard, practicing a little bit every day to improve their health, physical conditioning, and skills at martial arts. They should try to learn something new, no matter how small, from every person in every class.

Tradition

"The word dojo translated means "the place to learn the way," and Orientals consider it a valuable place of many lessons where a practitioner may learn to master himself as well as his opponent... He is also taught respect for those who make his practice and knowledge possible. Surely such a place deserves respect." [25]

– Dr. Hayward Nishioka Sensei
Pan-American Games Judo Gold Medalist, 1967,
US National Judo Champion, 1965, 1966, and 1970

It is very important to respect the traditions of our art. While boxing, wrestling, and other sports are frequently associated with name callers, ear biters, steroid abusers, and generally poor sportsmen (and women), Asian martial arts have managed to maintain their dignity. I believe the reason for this stems from an adherence to the traditions of these arts. It is important to learn the history and understand the basic terminology of whichever martial art one chooses to study.

An essential tradition is that there is no first strike in karate. It is practiced for physical conditioning, mental discipline, and self- defense purposes only. Clearly this helps practitioners of these lethal arts behave in a manner appropriate to interaction within polite society.

While it may seem odd to practice in "bare feet and pajamas," wearing the traditional *gi* in class is a very important tradition. It helps differentiate between training time and the rest of one's day, imparting essential focus. Although it is acceptable to travel from home to the *dojo*, or to training in one's *gi*, the *obi* (belt) should not be worn in public as it could very easily provoke confrontation with those predisposed toward violence in the first place. Bare feet help prolong the life of the *dojo* floor, protect against injury, and enhance the student's physical conditioning. There is nothing wrong, in my opinion, with practicing in street clothes outside the training hall, but *dojo* practice should always be traditional.

Although bowing is foreign to American culture, it is required in the *dojo* as a sign of respect toward the *dojo*, instructors, other students, and training equipment such as the *makiwara* (striking post) or *nigiri game* (gripping jars). American students may feel better knowing that bowing has no religious connotation but is a sign of mutual respect.

When we bow, both teacher and student say, "*Dozo one gaishimasu*," which means, "Please teach me," as both learn from each encounter. Similarly, at the end of training, both teacher and student say, "*Arigato gozaimashita*," which means, "Thank you for teaching me," as both have learned. These phrases are also said when bowing to other students before and after practicing together.

Dojo kun (virtues) are usually posted at the front of a *dojo*. They are recited either at the opening or the closing of class (or both) depending on the *dojo*. Members of the *dojo* recite the *kun* in hopes of making all those attending (or observing) better people in general, both physically and mentally. This ritual is meant to instill a positive ideal in each person hearing it.

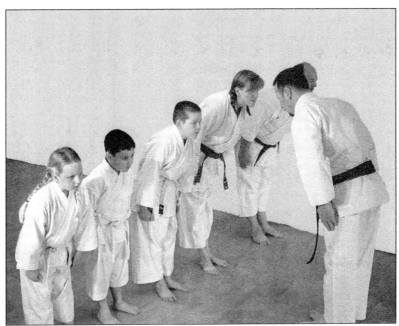

BOWING, IN AND OF ITSELF, HAS NO RELIGIOUS CONNOTATION IN MODERN MARTIAL ARTS; IT IS MERELY A SIGN OF MUTUAL RESPECT. *BUDOKA* TRADITIONALLY BOW TO EACH OTHER BEFORE AND AFTER PRACTICING TOGETHER. ETIQUETTE AND RESPECT ARE ESSENTIAL COMPONENTS OF *BUDO*.[G]

Although *dojo kun* tend to be similar within most *Goju Ryu* karate schools, the exact wording varies somewhat by instructor and system. *Dojo kun* are not numbered, as each item is equally important. We sometimes say *itos*, meaning first or most important, before each virtue.

Typically the most senior student in the class recites one line, which is then repeated by the entire class responsively until the progression is ended. In kids' classes, it is useful to have each of the senior students lead the recitation of one virtue where practicable. Through the practice of *budo*, the discipline of the body and mind, and the reciting of virtue we become better people, of higher nature, and better in contact with ourselves. The following *dojo kun* are used at the West Seattle Karate Academy:

We *karateka*:
- Respect good manners.
- Practice a sense of harmony.
- Learn to persevere.
- Give our minds to application.
- Make every effort to agree among heart and technique.
- As students, and later teachers, will follow the dojo rules.

Emotional Environment

"Traditional schools emphasize self-improvement and self-realization as the primary goal, with "not losing" (in an actual fight) a result of sincere training. Modern tournament schools emphasize being better than others, that is winning (and displaying) trophies. Fun is not the purpose of traditional karate-do; the development of good character is. To the extent that one has ego-centered fun at the expense of others, one has left the realm of self-improvement behind and sown the seeds of self-destruction. On the other hand, training cannot be distasteful. It has the rewards of happiness, fascination, satisfaction, and even humor, and it is on this feedback that the instructor and the club will succeed or fail." [26]

– Dr. Elmar T. Schmeisser Sensei, Godan
American Teacher's Association
of the Martial Arts (ATAMA)

Those who have a positive attitude and are willing to follow the rules and traditions of the art should always be made to feel welcomed by everyone in the *dojo*. Students may have no interest in social contact outside the training hall, and may not even particularly like each other, but they must be able to work harmoniously together to advance each other's training. Everyone truly needs to be able to trust and respect each other in order to feel confident practicing dangerous techniques and developing new skills in a supportive environment.

The etiquette and tradition inherent in most martial arts foster an environment of inclusion where *budoka* (martial artists) of all ages, races, religions, sexes, creeds, and other differences are able to train together in an atmosphere of trust and respect. Everyone in this fraternity of martial artists can and should be able to learn something new, no matter how small, from everyone else at every training session. Practitioners often come to view each other as partners in a lifelong learning process.

It is important to ensure that new students understand that there is no "can't" in martial arts. It is perfectly all right for students to state that they are "still working on it", "have not mastered it yet", or "are trying as best they can" as all of those sentiments reflect willingness and perseverance. It is not all right, on the other hand, to verbally or physically portray reluctance, vacillation, or defeat.

Possessing little natural athletic ability or inherent talent for martial arts myself, I have found that striving consistently is more important than aptitude. Through repetition and disciplined practice one can quickly build skill and confidence. For students to be successful, a spirit of resolve and determination must be instilled as early in their training as possible.

Physical Environment

"It is absolutely imperative that an instructor meditate deeply on the limits of his or her self control. Instructors who cannot prevent their tempers, emotions, or egos from asserting themselves on others in a malicious way pose a serious threat to students and threaten the success of their schools. Any lack of control, however slight, should be immediately aired out

*by talking or by vacating the area for a change of
scenery. Everyone has buttons that can be pushed.
Find out what your exploding point is and seek ways
to keep yourself calm under fire."* [27]

– Christopher J. Goedecke Sensei,
Director and Chief Instructor,
Wind School of Karate-Do

The first impression one receives upon entering a new *dojo*
will have a lasting impact on his or her perception of the instructor and the martial art. Training areas should be clean and neat,
with equipment and facilities in proper working order. There
should be adequate lighting and sufficient space for planned
activities. Strategically placed mirrors can facilitate intrinsic
feedback and self-correction during practice and are especially
valuable for visual learners. Practice areas should be as clear as
possible of obstructions, trip hazards, and sharp corners. If support pillars exist, they should be padded. Because most martial
artists practice in bare feet, it is a good idea to prohibit shoes in
the training area and to sweep or mop the floor daily. Practice
mats should routinely be cleaned with detergent or a bleach-
and-water solution when they get sweaty or bloody.

When children's classes are taught, it is very good to have
a separate viewing space where parents can comfortably and
safely watch their progeny without interfering with class activities. Encouraging this surveillance will greatly enhance parent's comfort level in allowing their children to participate in
what is often perceived as an inherently dangerous activity.

Physical safety in the *dojo* is paramount. No matter what
happens, *budoka* should always be in control of their techniques and never lose their tempers. Although most martial arts
require vigorous physical contact, students and teachers alike
should never intentionally injure anyone in class. Practitioners
should remove jewelry; keep their fingernails and toenails
short; be attentive to other practitioners; and carefully judge
range, speed, and distance to avoid accidentally hurting themselves or others.

Since instructors (and senior students) should have more patience, control, and understanding than those of lower ranks, they are always responsible for the physical safety of *both* participants in tandem practice situations. The higher belt always receives any attack first. That way the junior partner not only always knows what is expected of him or her, but has an opportunity to adequately prepare before his or her turn to defend against an attack.

In free sparring situations, vigilant oversight by senior instructors and members of the *dan* ranks is essential. Never let students (or teachers) simply beat up on each other. *Randori*

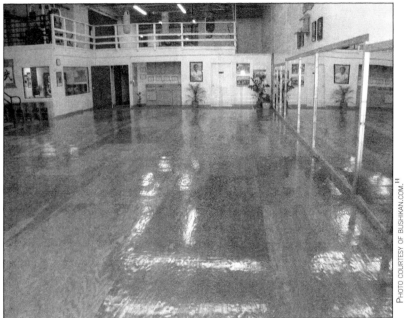

PHOTO COURTESY OF BUSHIKAN.COM.^H

THIS IS ONE OF THE BEST-DESIGNED *DOJOS* I HAVE SEEN. THE *SHOMEN* AT THE FRONT OF THE ROOM HAS BEEN RAISED HIGH ENOUGH THAT IT IS OUT OF THE WAY. TRADITIONAL AND MODERN WEIGHT TRAINING EQUIPMENT IS AVAILABLE ON THE UPPER BALCONY SO THAT THE WHOLE FLOOR REMAINS OPEN AND USABLE. MIRRORED WALLS FACILITATE VISUAL LEARNING. THERE IS A SEPARATE VIEWING ROOM AT THE FAR END WHERE VISITORS CAN COMFORTABLY OBSERVE WITHOUT INTERFERING. THE BACK WALL (NOT PICTURED HERE) IS LINED WITH TRADITIONAL *KOBUDO* WEAPONS SUCH AS *BO* AND *SAI* AND TRAINING EQUIPMENT SUCH AS *CHIISHI* AND *MAKIWARA*. DUMBBELLS AND OTHER EQUIPMENT SUCH AS *NIGIRI GAME* AND *ISHISASHI* ARE NEATLY STORED IN CUBBIES BY THE STAIRS.

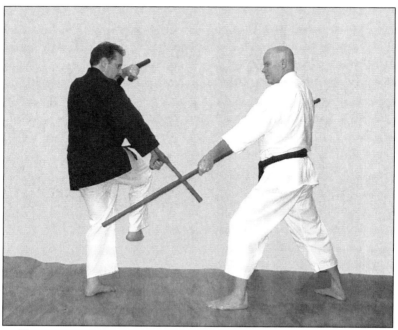

VIGILANCE IS ESPECIALLY IMPORTANT WITH WEAPONS TRAINING. *BUDOKA* PICTURED HERE PRACTICE WITH *TONFA* AND *BO*, TRADITIONAL *KOBUDO* WEAPONS, WITHOUT ANY PADDING OR PROTECTION WHATSOEVER. NOT ONLY MUST THEY RIGOROUSLY CONTROL THEIR TECHNIQUES TO AVOID SERIOUS INJURY OR DEATH, BUT THEY MUST ALSO BE CONSTANTLY AWARE OF THE CONDITION OF THEIR WEAPONS, WHICH, NO MATTER HOW WELL MADE, MAY BREAK ON OCCASION.[1]

facilitates a greater understanding of timing, distance, and control. However, if *budoka* are not practicing actual techniques (e.g., just throwing wild punches or kicks), they might as well be playing a game of tag. They will be missing valuable learning opportunities and can even be developing bad habits, which will ultimately get them seriously hurt in a real fight.

Regardless of instructor care and oversight, things occasionally do go wrong and someone gets hurt. All *dojos* must have appropriate first aid supplies readily available, including gloves to protect against blood-borne pathogens and bleach-water solution to decontaminate any fluid spills. To achieve higher *kyu* (colored belt) ranks, karate practitioners are typically required to obtain valid first aid/CPR certification. I wholeheartedly approve of this practice. All instructors should be familiar with emergency procedures and trained in both first aid and CPR (and Automated External Defibrillator [AED] where the defibrillator device is available).

Tailoring to Special Student Needs

"Someone had picked Kevin, a slight man in a wheelchair, as an easy target to rob. But when he tried to grab Kevin's waist bag, the attacker got the surprise of his life. The victim grabbed back. While pulling the robber forward and down with one hand, Kevin's other hand in a fist met the attacker in the face. By the time several people from a nearby store reached the pair, the attacker was on his back on the sidewalk with Kevin sitting over him, threatening to hit again.

"Kevin has taught me never to make quick judgments and never to underestimate someone. He has also taught me that each of us is very different and that each has his or her own strengths, weaknesses and goals. Karate helped him become stronger, better coordinated and helped him feel he could fit in and accomplish something he had set out to do. Being mostly a solo activity, karate thus proved to be an excellent form of physical therapy. And in Kevin's case it also helped him develop spirit and self-discipline. Perhaps it is something that more people with coordination and body control problems could benefit from . . ." [28]

– Christopher Caile Sensei, Rokudan

There is a community pool near our house where they have dedicated special classes with one-on-one instruction for blind children who wish to learn to swim. At Renton Technical College, I had deaf, blind, paraplegic, and quadriplegic students enroll in various computer classes, all of whom were able to successfully demonstrate required competencies and pass the course. While such individuals are not always attracted to the martial arts, it is important for instructors to think about which disabilities can reasonably be accommodated and which cannot.

Growing up, I had a neighbor who had lost both legs to a landmine during the Korean War. Though confined to a wheelchair, he continued to exercise regularly and had the largest arms I have ever seen (and having stood less than ten feet away from Governor Arnold Schwarzenegger, I do have an impressive reference for comparison). He also practiced martial arts and when I new him had reached the rank of *shodan* (though I suspect he is much higher than that by now, some 23 years later).

Although I do not remember which style he studied, my neighbor's *sensei* was able to modify techniques specifically to draw upon the strengths and minimize the weaknesses of his condition. For example, he learned how to remove the armrests from his wheelchair and use them like *tonfa* (a traditional Okinawan weapon similar to a modern police baton) to execute blocking and striking techniques. He also learned how to fight when lying on the ground without relying on his legs for support or movement.

Similarly, he was also able to bring new insight on the application of martial concepts back to his school. For example, he once taught a seminar on how to fight if someone is attacked when sitting on a toilet where one's legs are incapacitated by one's pants (the *samurai*, always ready to meet an attack, were actually taught to remove one pant leg to avoid becoming entangled when forced to fight in this situation). To ensure proper decorum, they actually practiced these techniques sitting on chairs, fully dressed, with their *obi*'s tied around their knees to limit leg movement. This example not only demonstrated effective techniques that might be used when confronted in an unusual situation, but also helped students recognize the obstacles and opportunities presented by various physical challenges.

Examples like these are not only inspirational, but they also portray how instructors can creatively tailor their art to accommodate special student needs and how individuals with such needs bring important diversity and perspective to the *dojos* where they study. Even when there are not current students that require special accommodations, it is prudent to prepare for such eventualities.

Exemplary Students, Exemplary Instructors

"It takes more than a flash of cash and sporadic attendance to succeed in a traditional dojo. Students must be considered worthy and dedicated by their instructor. More is expected of a Bugeisha (martial artist) than an ordinary person." [29]

– Dave Lowry

Dojos in feudal Japan were very selective. Gaining admission was an onerous process. Aspirants had to approach the *dojo* with letters of introduction and recommendation from someone well known to and respected by the head of the school. Far-reaching background checks were conducted on each candidate. When someone's application was accepted, they proceeded to swear a blood oath or *keppan* to guard the school's secrets and uphold the honor of the *ryu* (system). This loyalty oath was placed in writing then signed and sealed with the applicant's blood. Small scars on the inside of their arms (or sometimes their fingers) reminded them of the great honor it was to have been granted this opportunity.

Once the aspirant had sworn his oath and been accepted as a member of the *ryu*, the application was still not complete. A period of *hodoki* (unleashing or untying of the hands) followed where the applicant proved that he was worthy of training. During this probationary stage, he was given all manner of menial chores to perform (e.g., sweeping the floor, chopping wood, washing uniforms, preparing meals) as instructors tested how much the aspirant could tolerate to determine how badly he wanted to learn. If the beginner performed the assigned tasks with patience and perseverance, he could be inducted into the ranks of the *ryu*.

Once accepted, the student became a *monjin* (person at the gate), one who was eligible to actually begin their training. After this, it still took years of faithful service and vigorous effort before the student could learn, or even know about, the *okuden* (hidden teaching) or secret techniques of a school or martial style. In the old days, training was clearly more than simply attending lessons and picking-up new skills. *Budoka* were part of a privileged group who followed a life-long path toward becoming better people as well as highly skilled practitioners.

Today, anyone can pay an initiation fee, buy a uniform, and join almost any *dojo* in the country. Although there is no longer any *keppan* or formal *hodoki*, turnover rates among students being what they are, few instructors devote their full attention to new *budoka* until they have proven that they are worthy of such training. The rare student who demonstrates, discipline, perseverance, and a positive attitude will gradually be given access to more and more of the instructor's time, attention, and specialized guidance.

While a degree of instructor accommodation for student preferences is certainly necessary for effective learning, education is a two-way street. Teachers need to be able to recognize and nurture exemplary students just as students need to be able to recognize and adopt excellent instructors.

Characteristics of Exemplary Students

Through the practice of *budo*, the discipline of the body and mind, and the recitation of virtue we can become better people, of higher nature, and better in contact with ourselves. Many of the characteristics that describe exemplary students can be found in the *dojo kun* (see *Tradition*), good manners, inner harmony, perseverance, and following the rules, to name a few.

Character is important. Students approach martial arts for a plethora of reasons, some good, some bad, and many in-between. Because we teach our students dangerous, if not deadly techniques, the way in which they expect to use them is very important. I suspect that no instructor wants to be responsible for teaching some "hothead" what he or she needs to know to kill or maim another person in a drunken brawl.

Good manners among martial artists go beyond lip service to the traditions of bowing and etiquette. A judicious approach to using martial skills within and beyond the *dojo* must be applied. For example, students (or teachers for that matter) who like to "thump" on their juniors, start fights, or show off their skills in inappropriate manners should not be tolerated. We should always train together as partners, never as opponents.

Students who have good manners and respect the same in others are ideal, of course, but through proper coaching and discipline, recalcitrant individuals may be brought around as well. The question is whether or not they have enough moral fiber to make it worth your while. Revenue alone, in my opinion, is not sufficient reason to allow someone of questionable character to remain in class.

By inner harmony, I am in no way suggesting that the ideal student is currently meditating on a mountaintop somewhere waiting for you to arrive. I feel strongly, however, that balance between one's personal, professional, and educational priorities is important. Children need to finish their homework before they come to class, and should maintain good grades in their regular school if they wish to participate on a continuous basis. Even though *budo* provides a great deal of benefit, it should never be a child's first priority. Family and school must come first.

As adults, this balance is essential too. While daily training is an admirable quality, it should not be done at the expense of family, friends, school, or business commitments. This certainly should not preclude regular, intensive training, of course. It simply needs to harmoniously fit within a larger set of priorities.

In addition to working full-time, I have two part-time jobs one of which is seasonal, where I supervise security personnel at a Pac-10 football stadium. The other is teaching karate. Beyond that, I help my son with his schoolwork and karate practice, bring him to Scouting events, volunteer as the treasurer of his school's parent's club, and spend quality time with my wife. When I was asked to teach karate four nights a week rather than the current two, I had to respectfully decline. Although I am really devoted to teaching and would enjoy additional practice, there is just not enough time in the week for me to take on any additional responsibilities and still be able to guarantee that I can meet all my commitments.

Perseverance is essential to learning martial arts. The training is not easy. New students will find that they need to relearn how to perform basic functions they thought they understood such as moving and breathing. Exemplary students train every day, even if only for a few minutes. Consequently even the least athletic among them shows steady, continuous improvement in their techniques. In some ways perseverance is even more important for gifted athletes than it is for the rest of us. Naturally talented individuals are used to quick success and often lack the discipline necessary to push to the next level once they reach plateaus in their training.

There is also pain to work through, everything from minor bruises and strained muscles to the occasional serious injury. Back in my younger days, when I entered tournament competitions on a regular basis, I eventually needed surgery on both knees (at different times) due to cartilage damage. It would have been very easy to quit after a surgery, and even easier after two, but I worked my way back and now have stronger, more pain free knees than I did before I got hurt.

Dojo rules (see *Dojo Rules*) exist for a reason. Following such rules brings order to the learning process, facilitates safety, provides structure for training, and demonstrates a willingness to learn. A positive attitude is really essential. Disruptive individuals damage themselves and others. If students are unwilling to follow the rules once they understand them, they should not be allowed to participate.

Characteristics of an exemplary student include the following:

- A high degree of integrity, personal honor, and strong moral character.
- Willingness to ask questions and admit what he or she does not know.
- Enthusiasm to actively participate and learn.
- A sense of propriety and good manners, both inside and outside the *dojo*.

- A sense of harmony and balance among their priorities with the ability to meet all commitments.
- A strong work ethic.
- Ability to persevere.
- Desire share knowledge with others.

Nurturing Exemplary Students

Students who demonstrate good manners, practice a sense of harmony, show perseverance, have a positive attitude, and follow the rules should be rewarded. Such individuals show-up on time, work diligently, perform well, help others, and are a real asset to their class. Every reasonable effort should be exerted to motivate and retain them. This includes tailoring instruction to meet their personal preferences, of course, but it can go beyond that as well.

Motivation must be personality appropriate. Suggestions include encouraging perfection of skills through one-on-one coaching with instructors or senior students, broadening a student's knowledge through instructor training, offering membership on elite demonstration or competition teams, and providing opportunities to teach should a student be interested in doing so. Such individuals may be invited to special seminars or provided other mentoring opportunities not regularly available to all members of the class.

Our *dojo*, for example, focuses primarily on unarmed techniques. When I expressed interest in learning traditional weapons forms and my instructor thought I was ready, he introduced me to an affiliated *sensei* who was a black belt in *Goju Ryu* and also taught *kobudo* (a weapon-based martial system).

Finding an Exemplary Instructor

There are only a limited number of ways that each joint in the body can move. Similarly, there are only a limited number of vital areas on the body that can be manipulated, struck, or otherwise damaged. As much as we would like to think that our favorite martial art is unique and special, it undoubtedly shares components of other arts. Emphasis and strategies will

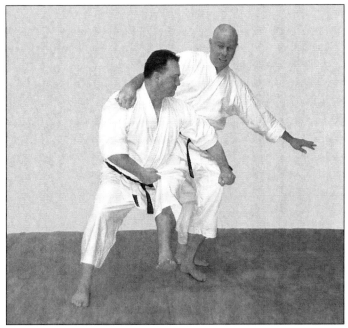

WHILE STRATEGIES AND EMPHASIS DIFFER, MOST *BUDO* STYLES SHARE COMMON TECHNIQUES. FOR EXAMPLE, JUDO AND KARATE UTILIZE MANY OF THE SAME THROWS. THE SCOOPING THROW, *SUKUI NAGE,* DEMONSTRATED HERE IS PART OF THE JUDO CURRICULA, YET IT IS ALSO FOUND IN *SEIYUNCHIN KATA* FROM *GOJU RYU* KARATE.[J]

differ, of course, but techniques always overlap.

For example, *tae kwon do* places great emphasis on kicking necessitating a different range (distance to the opponent) predilection than karate, which has a larger emphasis on strikes delivered with the hands. Regardless, both styles use front, side, back, and hook kicks. Judo and karate utilize many of the same throwing, grappling, and strangling techniques, though they are a much larger part of the judo curricula hence more of them are taught in that form than are taught in karate.

Tai chi metaphorically boils an egg from the inside out (with its emphasis on internal energy), while karate boils an egg from the outside in (as it starts with external power). Either way, you get a boiled egg. Advanced practitioners of both arts are able to harness both internal and external energy.

Because of this similarity and overlap, I have found that the teacher is more important to effective learning than the style

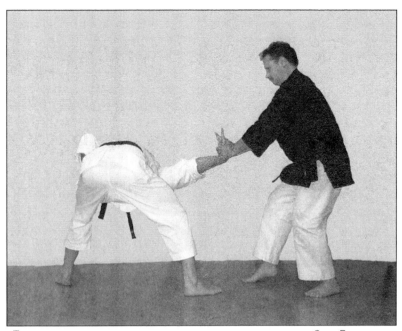

THE *NIKKYO* WRISTLOCK FROM AIKIDO IS ALSO FOUND IN *SAIFA KATA* FROM *GOJU RYU* KARATE. SINCE MANY MARTIAL SYSTEMS SHARE COMMON TECHNIQUES, THE TEACHER BECOMES MORE IMPORTANT TO EFFECTIVE LEARNING THAN STYLE BEING TAUGHT..[K]

being taught. New students should choose the art they wish to study in large part by choosing person who will be teaching it. No one should feel forced to learn from an instructor who does not fulfill his or her needs. Even experienced practitioners have a choice of *dojos* in which to continue practicing their current styles. Some may even choose to change styles based upon the caliber of instructor(s) they find. Several advanced practitioners in our school actually have black belts in other styles but have decided to train with us.

To find an exemplary instructor, first you need to determine why you are interested in martial arts in the first place. Are you looking for character development, tournament competition, physical conditioning, mental discipline, self-defense, weapons forms, any or all of the above, or something completely different?

Our interests in *budo* generally evolve and change over time. As children we may be drawn to martial arts simply because it is fun. Building strength, balance and coordination are definite benefits, as is a sense of accomplishment as we overcome challenges, receive promotions, and enhance our self-esteem. Our parents likely appreciate the discipline and conditioning aspects more than we do. As young adults, however, we may be more concerned with the combat or tournament aspects of our art. Social interactions and physical conditioning are also a draw. As we reach our late 30s or early 40s, however, many practitioners begin looking for something deeper, such as internal (*ki*) training, character development, or even spiritual enlightenment.

Once you know what you are looking for, you will need to find an instructor who can meet those needs. The best source, of course, is a referral by someone who knows you well, understands how you learn, and also knows someone appropriate who teaches martial arts. If you do not have friends or relatives who can refer you to an excellent instructor, however, you can start you search by looking in the Yellow Pages for you local area or conducting an online search. Make a list of *dojos* nearby, visit them, interview the instructors to get a feel for their methods, and ask if you can observe a class.

A good initial approach is to ascertain the emphasis of each *dojo*. Much of this can be understood simply by walking through the door. Schools whose front windows are crowded with trophies most likely have an emphasis on tournament fighting and competition. The presence of pads and headgear may reinforce this initial impression. Depending upon you age and interests, this may or may not be attractive. Stacks of *tatami* or other practice mats indicate a propensity for grappling techniques. Racks of weapons offer an obvious clue. The presence of *kigu undo* equipment (traditional tools used for conditioning exercises such as *chiishi* and *makiwara*) suggests a traditional approach, one that bodes well if your goal is character development.

Beyond the obvious, however, you can tell a lot about how a school is run by looking across the *dojo* floor during a class. Are students standing around looking confused or does everyone appear to be actively engaged in the learning process? Are they talking or working? Do students and teachers interact in a respectful manner? Are students corrected in a positive way when they make a mistake? Is there proper supervision?

If the *dojo* rules and/or *dojo kun* are posted on the wall, does what they say make sense to you? Are students training in traditional uniforms or modern street clothes? Assuming shoes are not worn during class, are they lined-up neatly in front of the floor? Is the place neat, orderly, and in good repair? Is there a viewing area where parents can observe their children without getting in the way? Is there adequate room to train? Does there appear to be an appropriate emphasis on safety? Is attendance strong?

Once you have made a preliminary decision, many *dojos* offer one or more free classes to help you decide whether or not training there will be right for you. It really takes a minimum of two to three months to know for sure (especially if you have not done this sort of thing before), but much can be intuited with a single class. I would not personally join any school that did not give me a *minimum* of at least one trial class.

Be wary of large initiation fees or long-term contracts. Some instructors whose only source of income is teaching martial arts may use unscrupulous or manipulative tactics to bring revenue through the door. Month-to-month arrangements are best. Requirements to pay a moderate initiation fee and purchase a uniform are perfectly reasonable. Even if you already have a uniform, if it is not the same type as that used by the rest of the class you can expect to be required to purchase a new one.

While there are a variety of online sources for purchasing *gi's*, most schools can provide them for you at a reasonable cost. They can also help with sizing or tailoring when needed. Uniforms are generally sized numerically in a fashion that does not correlate with any other method of clothing dimensions. Online conversion tables do not always account for shrinkage accurately.

If properly approached, teachers should be happy to discuss their styles, testing methodologies, and teaching approaches with prospective students. Be respectful of their time, however, preparing questions ahead of time and making an appointment when necessary. Just as you are forming an initial impression of a potential instructor, your future *sensei* is forming his or her impression of you.

Instructors need to be firm yet polite when disciplining students, informative when explaining new skills, and persuasive when teaching the more esoteric aspects of their art. They should be approachable for answering questions and polite no matter how silly the questions might be. Above all else, exemplary educators are always prepared and ready to teach each class in a professional manner.

After interviewing an instructor, it may be possible to talk with students and/or parents of students to gather more information. Exemplary instructors have nothing to hide and should not mind such additional scrutiny so long as it is not disruptive to their students.

Characteristics of an exemplary instructor include following:

- A high degree of integrity, personal honor, and strong moral character.
- Enthusiasm for practicing the chosen martial art
- A passion for teaching.
- A deep, well rounded knowledge of *budo*, preferably beyond a single art form.
- A high degree of perception regarding the needs and interests of students.
- A good understanding of personality differences among students and a demonstrated willingness to accommodate them as necessary.
- An intuitive ability to select the most effective teaching style for any situation and a willingness to change course midstream if things are not working as anticipated.
- Ability to communicate a sense of direction and purpose for his or her school and art form.
- An open mind, tempered with a great deal of common sense.

Teacher/Student Relationships

The relationship between student and teacher is complex, especially in the field of martial arts where instructors may hold a higher-degree of power over their students than in other disciplines. While a math or science teacher can flunk you, manipulate you, threaten you, or otherwise mess up your life, he or she works for an institution with strict bylaws, governance, and oversight. If a student's professor does something inappropriate, there is generally a review board and dispute process to follow.

A *budo* instructor, on the other hand, can kill you. Furthermore, he or she often runs his or her own school with limited, if any, oversight by an association of that style. Consequently such relationships need to be deeply founded on trust, integrity, and honesty, untainted by even the appearance of impropriety.

Most *budo* instructors will distance themselves, at least a little, from all but the most senior, dedicated students. Thought not as formalized as the old days, modern *senseis* will typically not go out of their way to provide "secrets" or special assistance to those who have not proven themselves over a significant period of time. That is just human nature.

Additionally, there is a certain degree of professionalism and detachment that is prudent when interacting with students. We live in a highly litigious society where even an unfounded accusation of harassment or sexual misconduct can ruin one's reputation and livelihood.

Because instructors have a great deal of power, both real and perceived, over their students, it is important to separate personal and professional relationships. Teachers should be leery of discussing any personal matters in the *dojo*, even if some of their students are friends on the outside. Tribulations in one's personal life simply do not belong on the *dojo* floor.

While intimate relationships between teachers and students should be strictly taboo, dating between equals in the *dojo* can be somewhat less restrictive. Practitioners often develop deep interpersonal bonds based on years of training closely together. So long as personal issues are kept from interfering with the smooth operation of the *dojo*, such relationships should not be discouraged. Although we have had several occasions where dating and/or married partners trained together with no problems, if couples broke up one party or the other invariably stopped training at our *dojo*.

Friends and family members often train together as well. Once again, great care must be taken to ensure that personal issues are kept outside the *dojo*. For example, my son is one of my students. I'm probably a little tougher on him than on his fellow students yet, I strive very hard to ensure that there is no favoritism. He understands that while I might be "dad" everywhere else, in the *dojo*, I'm "*sensei.*" To avoid even the appearance of impropriety, I have arranged for another instructor to handle my son's advancement and testing. Should my wife ever decide to practice karate, I would handle her education in much the same way.

Dojo relationship guidelines:

- Keep all interactions professional, positive, and *budo*-related; avoid discussing personal matters in the *dojo*.
- Never date your students—while there is certainly an upside if things work out well (e.g. marriage, happily ever after, and all that good stuff), it may cause distraction, resentment, or litigation, and will frequently end badly.
- If a family member is one of your student's, segregate the personal and professional relationship to the extent possible, making great efforts to avoid even the appearance of favoritism or impropriety (e.g., arranging for another instructor to handle the testing and advancement).
- When touching students, especially children, ensure that it is done in plain sight.
- Always have more than one person in the room when working with members of the opposite sex.
- Know your limitations—resist the temptation to be a priest, counselor, or psychologist for your students.

Summary

The general mindset and biases of the students with whom teachers plan to share information will color what they can hear and how they hear it. These biases are both intellectual as well as emotional. Influences on how people will interpret what is presented include their previous experience with and attitude about the subject matter, what is urgent and important to them at the time of instruction, the mental models through which they make sense of the world, any previous experience they might have had (or may have heard about) with the instructor, and any outside issues that may distract their attention.

The instructor's attitude is paramount to effective communication. Martial arts are competency based, not letter graded along a curve. When educators truly believe that their primary role is to impart knowledge, they will be motivated to creatively find appropriate mechanisms that ensure their students will learn. Remember to consider that when a student does not understand a lesson, it is almost always the teacher's fault.

Etiquette is an integral part of martial arts, for without it we would be practicing nothing more than base violence. The primary emphasis of most martial arts is on character development of the *budoka* themselves rather than on merely training for tournaments or sports competition. While competition has its place, such activities must fit within a much larger context.

Everyone needs to be able to trust and respect each other in order to feel confident that they can practice dangerous techniques and develop new skills in a supportive environment. Instructors can creatively tailor their arts to accommodate the needs of special students. These individuals often bring important diversity and perspective to the *dojos* where they study. Even when there are not current students that require special accommodations, it is wise to preplan for such eventualities.

Today, anyone can pay an initiation fee, buy a uniform, and join almost any *dojo* in the country. Turnover rates among students being what they are, however, few instructors will devote their full attention to new *budoka* until they have proven that they are worthy of such training. The rare student who demonstrates, discipline, perseverance, and a positive attitude will gradually be given access to more and more of the instructor's time, attention, and specialized guidance. Teachers need to be able to recognize and nurture exemplary students just as students need to be able to recognize and adopt excellent instructors.

CHAPTER 5

✴ Dojo Lesson Planning ✴

"In terms of structuring the individual class time, I generally run formal warm-up exercises only for the first month or so of the new semester. Thereafter the students are expected to arrive sufficiently early that they are warmed up and stretched out at the class starting time. Auxiliary strengthening exercises are also left to the student. I prefer to spend as much time on actual karate training as possible, following the theory that practice produces improvement only on what is practiced—that is, pushups are not punches." [30]

– Dr. Elmar T. Schmeisser Sensei

Formal lesson planning is a great enabler for successful seminars and other short-term classes. It is also quite useful in continuous learning applications, as individual class sessions can be arranged to facilitate skill development commensurate with advancement requirements (see *Testing and Advancement Principles*).

Such planning consists of the following:

- Creating skill/knowledge statements.
- Forming program objectives.
- Developing course outlines.
- Choosing appropriate instructional methods to accomplish these goals.

Skill/knowledge statements describe what the student must be able to do and/or know how to perform effectively. A common example of this type would be a list of advancement requirements promulgated for each rank (see *Advancement Requirement Essentials Table*). Because martial arts are competency based, such requirements should be as objective and measurable as possible.

Program objectives express an intended goal for the overall curriculum and the necessary conditions that must be met to achieve that outcome. They also document the standard by which success or failure will be measured in a specific and observable manner. A formal *course outline*, on the other hand, lists specific objectives that must be accomplished in a subordinated list, including lesson and enabling objectives that must be reached along the path toward achieving the terminal or final course objective.

Individual lessons should be approached within a "Plan–Do–Check–Act" framework, allowing for optimal utilization of teacher/student interaction and classroom time management.

At one extreme, the planning phase may be done with great rigor and detail prior to commencement of class sessions. At the other, planning may be done during *daruma* (warm-up exercises) just before the beginning of formal instructions. Regardless of the level and forethought, sufficient planning must be performed to assure a reasonable progression from one subject to another throughout each training session. Once planning is completed, training may commence.

During the "do" phase, the plan is executed. Progress must be monitored to ensure that the class is moving forward commensurate with the plan, and that the original plan still has merit once actual interaction with students occurs. While the military principle of no plan surviving initial contact with the enemy would be an inappropriate analogy, in any classroom environment things inevitably do go wrong. Your best-laid plans simply will not work right every time.

To paraphrase Will Rogers, when you find yourself in a hole, the first thing you want to do is stop digging. If a check shows that the plan is not working, stop. Adjust the plan accordingly then proceed with a modified lesson, hence the "act" phase. Obviously when things go well the appropriate act is continuance of the original plan.

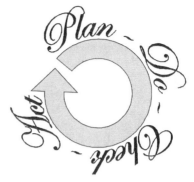

FIGURE 3. THE PLAN-DO-CHECK-ACT CYCLE.

This Plan–Do–Check–Act cycle should be repeated throughout each class session. When plans go awry, as they frequently do, this context allows an instructor to exercise his or her creativity and flexibility to make in-course corrections without undue panic, stress, or wasted time.

Formal Plans for Individual Lessons

Once you have created skill/knowledge statements, formed program objectives, developed course outlines, and selected appropriate instructional methods to accomplish these goals, you may wish to formally document plans for some or all of the individual lessons. This is especially beneficial for newer instructors who may be uncomfortable conducting planning on the fly. In many cases, senior instructors or administrators have already developed lesson plans that new instructors must initially follow and will later customize after gaining experience.

Formal lesson plan formats usually have most or all of the following elements:

- Content
- Prerequisites
- Instructional objectives
- Instructional procedures
- Materials or equipment listing

- Evaluation process
- Follow-up activities
- Self-assessment

Content is the concept or skill to be taught during the lesson. The depiction of concept-oriented content is generally written as "students will understand [description]." Skill-oriented content is commonly described as "students will be able to do [description]." Individual lesson content may include concepts, skills, or both.

Prerequisites are the knowledge or skills students must already have successfully learned before beginning the lesson. In other words, if they do not have certain specific knowledge, skills, or abilities, they will be unable to complete the lesson. I have found that more than half of what a student actually internalizes is predicated upon possessing the appropriate prerequisites. This is important when developing lesson plans for classes with mixed skill-levels, especially where several ranks separate beginning and advanced practitioners. In such cases, students may be given different learning objectives and instructional procedures according to rank or background.

Instructional objectives are what the individual students will do to demonstrate competency in the content they have been taught. There should be specific behavioral expectations in the objective such as passing a test or demonstrating a skill.

Instructional procedures are the specifics of how the lesson will be introduced, taught, and brought to closure. Keep the Plan–Do–Check–Act cycle in mind, developing fallback procedures in case things go awry.

The **materials or equipment listing** describes all equipment needed by teachers and students and how it will be used to further the instructional objective. It is a good idea to inventory training equipment on a regular basis to ensure that instructors know what is available and that everything is in working order.

Evaluation process describes how to determine the extent to which students have obtained the instructional objective. It must be tied to the behavioral expectations of the plan. Evaluations may be formal or informal (see *Testing and*

Advancement Principles). This process not only gauges student progress, but also may highlight inadequacies in an instructor's approach (e.g., particularly when the vast majority of students are making the same mistake).

Follow-up activities are other activities or materials that can be used to reinforce or extend the lesson. This may include outside homework assignments or other projects.

Self-assessment is completed after the lesson has been presented. In the Plan–Do–Check–Act cycle this is another form of check. Address all the major components of the lesson plan to identify areas of strength as well as those that need improvement. Just as a teacher's skills will progress over time, lesson plans should be continuously updated and improved. If they end up as "shelfware," there is little point in taking the time and energy required to create them (though you will gain some benefit simply from writing down ideas and methods—see *Knowledge Capture*). Appendix D provides a demonstration of how to create a lesson plan.

Classroom Management

> *"Student misbehavior isn't just an annoying disruption—it's a secret message the student is (unwittingly) trying to convey to you. And usually that message can be boiled down to two words: Reach Me!"* [31]
>
> – Dr. Tom Daly, author
> and teaching consultant

Teaching martial arts is a fairly serious business. Instructors must balance the somber reality that they are responsible for ensuring the safety of practitioners who learn potentially deadly techniques with the truism that should the training not be enjoyable, no one will participate in it. On the one hand instructors must ensure that students follow appropriate rules and decorum and adhere to essential etiquette and tradition. On the other, to the extent possible, teachers should sanction appropriate humor and camaraderie in the training. Above all, they must be in command of their classrooms at all times.

In a well-managed *dojo*, students are actively engaged in instructor-led activities or self-directed practice at all times. Not only do they know what they are expected to do, but teaching styles have been thoughtfully selected and communication techniques appropriately tailored such that they are generally successful at doing it. Students feel that they are making progress daily, learning something new, no matter how small, at each training session. There is little to no time wasted due to confusion or disruption. A work-oriented tone prevails, but within a relaxed, pleasant atmosphere.

The instructor's voice is an excellent tool for maintaining necessary control, especially when dealing with children. Commands should be given in a calm but crisp manner, using declarative language whenever possible. While a drill-instructor analogy may be a bit overstated, the spirit is essentially the same (e.g., *sensei* is "large and in charge," but without all the negative yelling, name-calling, foul language, and smelly cigars).

During the "Plan–Do–Check–Act" cycle, instructors can determine what they intend to say beforehand, facilitating required assertiveness and clarity. For example, rather than saying, "I think we should spend some time working on *kata*," the instructor should proclaim, "we will work on *gekisai kata dai ichi* now."

The energy of the room is highly affected by the instructor's choice of language and presentation. When a student's concentration wanders, the instructor's voice is an exceptional way to bring that student back to attention. During *daruma*, for example, counting louder and crisply can focus attention and step up the pace. Changes in tone, pitch, pacing, or volume may provide needed emphasis to reinforce a teacher's points. When used with appropriate timing, quiet words can sometimes be even more effective than loud ones.

Dojo Rules

The *dojo* rules must be clear and have a definite purpose. Disciplinary measures must be consistently and fairly applied.

When dealing with children, parental acceptance is an essential ingredient as well. Students should always be taught the *dojo* rules as part of their acclimation process upon joining a new class. When correcting a student, it is critical to focus on the student's behavior rather on him or her personally. Nothing positive ever comes from attacking or embarrassing someone in public.

Wayward students can be dissuaded from inappropriate behaviors through coaching sessions or various age and incident-appropriate penalties such as push-ups, cleaning the *dojo*, or writing a paper on the *dojo* rules and why they are important. At times interruptions are minor and it is more beneficial to focus on continuing the flow of the class rather than on correcting the errant student. It is important, however, to speak to the offending student after class so that your lack of action does not reinforce negative behaviors.

A blend of positive and negative reinforcement can be very effective. In addition to correcting inappropriate behavior through various disciplinary measures, students should actively be encouraged toward appropriate behaviors through positive incentives such as advancement, invitation to seminars, or ability to train one-on-one with senior students or teachers. Some schools formalize such reinforcement by holding annual barbeques or banquets where awards are presented for attendance, perseverance, improvement, and so on. Student of the month awards are also common.

Ensuring Appropriate Pacing

Most classes contain a mix of beginning, intermediate, and advanced students. Within those categories, some people inherently learn faster than others. It is important to pace the class toward the average student while providing challenging opportunities for the gifted and more experienced.

Exceptional students should be afforded knowledge and materials to improve more independently while additional help may be necessary for the slower learners. This balance is key. If the class is paced toward the slower learners, a majority of the students will become bored and uninterested. If it is paced toward the most gifted students, the majority will be lost and frustrated. It is often useful to present core curricula to the whole class and then break out small groups to work independently on materials appropriate to each group's level of knowledge and skill. It is also important to challenge each student to practice a little bit every day outside of class.

Testing and Advancement Principles

"Remember rank belts are used to bring order to the dojo, assist in training, show merit for hard work, and keep your gi closed." [32]

– *Kris Wilder Sensei, Yodan*

The founder of judo, Professor Jigoro Kano, codified a system of wearing colored sashes or belts, which was subsequently adopted by most martial arts systems and is widely used today. This *dan/kyu* system distinguishes between advanced practitioners and different levels of beginning and intermediate students. The *dan*, or black belt, indicates advanced proficiency. Those who have earned it are called *yudansha* (*dan* recipients). The *kyu* degrees represent the varying levels of competency below *dan*, and are called *mudansha* (those not yet having received a *dan* rank).

Kano *Sensei* felt it particularly important for all students to fully realize that one's training was in no way complete simply because they had achieved the *dan* degree. On the contrary, he emphasized that the attainment of the *dan* rank merely symbolized the real beginning of one's training. By reaching black belt level, one had, in fact, completed only the necessary requirements to embark upon a relentless expedition, a journey without distance that would ultimately result in self-mastery.

After establishing the *Kodokan Dojo*, Kano *Sensei* distributed black sashes, which were worn around the standard *dogi* (training uniform) of that era, to all *yudansha*. Around 1907, this black sash was replaced with the *kuroi-obi* (black belt), which became the standard that is still used today. Of this standard there was the white belt and the black belt. Later addition of green and brown belts rounded out the traditional ranking system.

By following a structure of merit, such as the belt system, instructors have a way of monitoring the development and skill progression of their students and can teach them according to set standards. *Goju Ryu* karate uses five *kyu* belts, white, yellow, green, blue, and brown, and three *dan* belts, black, *akashiro* (red/white), and red. Colored stripes on both ends of a *kyu* belt delineate gradations between *mudansha* ranks (some schools use additional colored belts, such as orange or purple, rather than colored-stripes to show these gradations). These stripes take the color of the next level of advancement such that white belts have yellow stripes, yellow belts have green stripes, green belts have blue stripes, blue belts have brown stripes, and brown belts have black stripes. In Okinawa, one or more gold stripes at the ends of a black belt indicate *shogo* (teaching degree) rank.

Training objectives must be stated in terms specific enough that students will know whether or not they have been accomplished (see *Advancement Requirements Table*). Evaluations must be well planned ahead of time, and instructors must be willing to act upon results. Continuous feedback is essential such that students will understand how they are progressing and are able to identify deficient areas upon which they should focus their training. This approach sets them up to succeed when advancement testing occurs.

Such feedback needs to be metered however so that it will not be overwhelming. When working with beginners it is a good idea to correct no more than three or four items per training session. As students advance and instructors begin to understand their personalities and learning styles, additional fine-tuning may be added as appropriate.

Formal versus Informal Testing

There are two philosophies for testing: formal and informal. With formal testing, time is set-aside for students to demonstrate skill requirements under the watchful eye of their instructors and the rest of the class. Typically one class session every quarter would be used for such activity. A short promotion ceremony would follow to advance those who pass the requirements. With informal testing, on the other hand, instructors monitor student performance over time and promote them once they have met the expected level of proficiency as appropriate. While testing among the *mudansha* ranks may be either formal or informal, testing in the *yudansha* ranks is often formalized, especially at the *shodan* level when a practitioner initially advances into the *dan* ranks.

Formal testing has been used as a revenue generation mechanism by certain *dojos* making it inherently unpalatable for some martial artists. It also runs the risk of leading practitioners into a "cram-for-finals" mentality where they practice hard right before testing and then slack off afterward. Informal testing, on the other hand, can facilitate a more holistic approach where practitioners are encouraged to do their best every day in each class with advancements awarded whenever appropriate. This approach is arguably more traditional as well.

A good analogy might be traveling from one place to another by bus versus car. Like formal testing, the bus follows prescribed routes and stops along the way. If it arrives at one stop too early, it will wait before proceeding. If it is running behind, it will attempt to catch up. The car, on the other hand, can travel by whatever path the driver wishes to follow. While the journey is somewhat different, you get to your destination either way. Although instructors should keep student personality types and learning style predilections in mind when determining whether to choose a formal or informal testing methodology, they must select one method or the other to follow. However, one may legitimately select a different option for *kyu* testing than for *dan* testing. I prefer informal testing for *kyu* ranks and formal testing for *dan* ranks where judges beyond an individual's school are often involved.

Validation and Reinforcement

Whether one chooses a formal or informal approach, however, testing should always be conducted in a way that is not

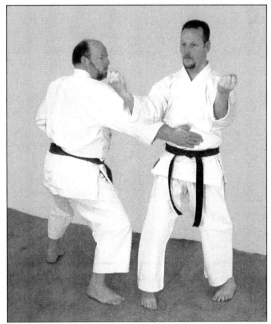

THE GOAL OF TESTING SHOULD ALWAYS BE VALIDATION AND REINFORCEMENT. *SANCHIN SHIMÉ* TESTING IS AN EXCELLENT EXAMPLE OF THIS APPROACH, AS GIVING PRESSURE AND STRIKING VARIOUS PARTS OF A KARATEKA'S BODY TESTS FOR FUNDAMENTALS SUCH AS CONCENTRATION, BODY ALIGNMENT, MOVEMENT, AND BREATHING. SLAPS AND KICKS SHOULD BE FIRM BUT NEVER DAMAGING.[L]

designed to embarrass or degrade participants. Instructors should not encourage students to participate in any public formal testing unless they have already progressed to a point where they have an extremely good chance to succeed. Furthermore, testing should never be designed to injure or humiliate students.

Done properly, *sanchin shimé* (testing of technique and power) testing is an excellent example of the proper approach to student evaluations. The way it works is that students complete *sanchin kata* while an instructor checks their concentration, body alignment, movement, breathing, and mechanics of their technique by giving pressure and striking various parts of the student's body. The teacher's slaps and kicks should be firm but never damaging as they provide essential validation and reinforcement.

Rank Number	Rank Name	Belt	Belt Color	Stripe Color	Number of Stripes	Min. Time in Prior Rank
10th Kyu	Jyu Kyu		White	None	N/A	N/A
9th Kyu	Kyu Kyu		White	Yellow	1	3 Months
8th Kyu	Hachi Kyu		Yellow	None	0	3 Months
7th Kyu	Shichi Kyu		Yellow	Green	1	3 Months
6th Kyu	Ro Kyu		Green	None	0	3 Months
5th Kyu	Go Kyu		Green	Blue	1	3 Months
4th Kyu	Yon Kyu		Blue	None	0	3 Months
3rd Kyu	San Kyu		Blue	Brown	1	6 Months
2nd Kyu	Ni Kyu		Brown	None	0	6 Months
1st Kyu	I Kyu		Brown	Black	1	6 Months
1st Dan	Shodan		Black	N/A	N/A	1 Year
2nd Dan	Nidan		Black	N/A	N/A	2 Years
3rd Dan	Sandan		Black	N/A	N/A	3 Years
4th Dan	Yodan		Black	N/A	N/A	4 Years
5th Dan	Godan		Black	N/A	N/A	5 Years
6th Dan	Roku dan		Akashiro	N/A	N/A	6 Years
7th Dan	Shichidan		Akashiro	N/A	N/A	7 Years
8th Dan	Hachidan		Akashiro	N/A	N/A	8 Years
9th Dan	Kudan		Red	N/A	N/A	9 Years
10th Dan	Judan		Red	N/A	N/A	10 Years

TABLE 3. RANKS AND ASSOCIATED BELT COLORS USED IN GOJU RYU KARATE.

Using the whole body to focus internal power rather than "separating" the body in a manner that forces reliance on brute muscle strength is a key aspiration of many Okinawan karate styles. *Shimé* testing helps practitioners focus on parts of the body that are not actively being used so that they do not forget about them, facilitating a practitioner's ability to concentrate on their whole body simultaneously. The force of the instructor's blows must be commensurate with the strength and skill of the person being tested.

Minimum Time in Rank Requirements

Most systems have minimum time requirements between each rank. While it is possible after four years of studying *Goju Ryu karate* to obtain a *shodan* rank, separation between *dan* ranks are based on years equivalent to the next rank. For example, the minimum time between the first *dan* rank, *shodan*, and the second *dan* rank, *nidan*, is two years (*nidan* = 2nd degree). The minimum time between *nidan*, the second *dan* rank, and *sandan*, the third *dan* rank, is three years (*san* is 3rd degree). So to go from *shodan* (1st degree) to *sandan* (3rd degree) takes a minimum of five (2+3) years (typically a lot longer unless you are truly a gifted athlete who has a lot of time to train). *Akashiro* (red/white) and red belts are reserved for the

Rank	Required *Kata* and *Kata Bunkai*	Other Requirement(s)
9th Kyu	Taikyoku Gedan	
8th Kyu	Taikyoku Chudan	
7th Kyu	Taikyoku Jodan	Te Waza Dai Ichi
6th Kyu	Gekisai Kata Dai Ichi and Bunkai	Goshin Do Ippon Kumite
5th Kyu	Gekisai Kata Dai Ni and Bunkai	Goshin Do Ippon Kumite
4th Kyu	Saifa Kata and Bunkai Sanchin Kata	Goshin Do Ippon Kumite
3rd Kyu	Seyunchin Kata and Bunkai	Goshin Do Ippon Kumite
2nd Kyu	Seisan Kata and Bunkai	Goshin Do Ippon Kumite
1st Kyu	Saipai Kata and Bunkai Tensho Kata	Goshin Do Ippon Kumite
Shodan	Shishochin Kata and Bunkai	Goshin Do Ippon Kumite Thesis
Nidan	Kurunfa Kata and Bunkai	Goshin Do Ippon Kumite Thesis
Sandan	Sanseiru Kata and Bunkai Suparinpei Kata and Bunkai	Goshin Do Ippon Kumite Thesis

TABLE 4. HOKUSEI YUDANSHAKAI ADVANCEMENT REQUIREMENTS

highest ranks and are rarely seen. These belts represent lifetime achievements and are worn by individuals who have devoted their lives to karate.

Using the minimum time between ranks formula, a *karate-ka* who started training at age twenty would be eligible for *roku dan*, the first red/white belt at age forty-five. *Ju dan*, the highest rank attainable, could happen somewhere around age seventy.

Advancement Essentials Table

The following table outlines essential advancement requirements for each rank through *sandan* (by which time the entire curricula has been completed). There are a number of basic techniques (e.g., stances, blocks, strikes, kicks, chokes, holds, throws) and miscellaneous requirements (e.g., time in rank, attendance, knowledge of Japanese words and phrases, *dojo* etiquette, first aid/CPR certification) related to the *kata, bunkai* and knowledge base required for each rank (see appendix A— *Hokusei Yudanshakai* Advancement Requirements for more details).

Progression of Class Activities

"Goju Ryu Karate-do is a manifestation within one's own self of the harmonious accord of the universe." [33]

– *Chojun Miyagi Sensei*

Classes should progress through a logical order that both assists in communication and facilitates efficient use of available time. Typically sessions begin with *mokuso* (meditation), proceed through *daruma* warm-up and sometimes *kigu hojo undo* (conditioning with traditional equipment) exercises prior to beginning work on actual martial technique.

From there, the class may build from *kihon* (basics) to *kata*, or start from *kata* and drill-down to application. Alternatively, the instructor may choose to focus all the remaining class time on a special, session-specific theme (e.g., break-fall techniques, self-defense, grappling techniques, or sparring). Regardless of the details, variety is imperative to maintaining student energy and interest.

Sessions should always begin with a brief meditation to set an appropriate mood and allow students to focus on their training without outside distraction. To avoid injury, warm-up exercises must precede strenuous physical activity. This may be done following the meditation, or it may be required of students to be completed on their own time prior to initiation of formal classroom training. Because form precedes speed and both form and speed are necessary to achieve power, basic techniques (e.g., stances, movement, kicks, punches, blocks, breathing) must be practiced repeatedly, yet not exclusively.

While training should focus more on the needs of the students than on those of the instructor, teachers cannot be everywhere at once. Successful instructors practice effective delegation. When students interact with and coach each other, they develop deeper understanding of the techniques they attempt to communicate and may also form friendships and camaraderie that extends beyond the *dojo*. Additionally, they get invaluable preparation for becoming instructors themselves and should take advantage of opportunities to practice their teaching and communication skills.

Opening and Closing Ceremonies

Each training session should begin and end with a short ceremony to show respect for the head instructor, any guest instructors, the *dojo*, and fellow students. This helps set the tone for the rest of the class. Although such ceremonies vary widely by school and art form, I have used an example from *Goju Ryu* karate to demonstrate how it works. Opening and Closing Ceremonies used in our *dojo* are described in Tables 5 and 6.

Teaching Daruma

"Strength and flexibility can be improved with karate practice with the concomitant advantage of learning technique, but strengthening and stretching exercises do not necessarily teach karate." [34]

– Dr. Elmar T. Schmeisser Sensei

In addition to always warming up before practicing, it is essential that students know their physical condition and practice accordingly. Proper hydration and breathing are also important. Whether students complete *daruma* on their own or as a group, instructors must ensure that everyone knows how to perform the exercises properly. Stretching should be completed both before *and* after strenuous physical activity.

	Who	What	Explanation
1.	Instructor	claps twice	Line up (Shugo)
2.	Head student	"Ki o tsuke"	Attention
3.	Head student	"Seiza"	Sit in kneeling stance
4.	Head student	"Mokuso hajime"	Close eyes/begin meditation
5.	Instructor	"Mokuso yame"	Open eyes/end meditation
6.	Head student	"Shomen ni"	Face forward (towards the Shomen)
7.	Head student	"Rei"	Bow (right hand forward first followed by left, then bow)
8.	Head student	"Sensei ni"	Face toward the instructor.
9.	Head student	"Rei"	Bow
10.	Everybody	"Dozo one gaishimasu"	Please teach me.
11.	Head student	"Yudansha ni"	Face toward the black belts or guest instructor(s), if any
12.	Head student	"Rei"	Bow
13.	Everybody	"Dozo one gaishimasu"	Please teach me
14.	Head student	"Shomen ni"	Face front
15.	Instructor	"Tatsu"	Straighten (stand up)

TABLE 5. OPENING CEREMONY

Exercises should always begin with jumping jacks, cross-marches (alternately raising right leg/left arm and vice versa), or other light aerobic activity to warm and loosen students' muscles such that stretching will not cause injury. A good analogy might be to think of the muscles as fresh cabbage leaves. When cold, they tear easily. Once warmed (e.g., by blanching in hot water), they become much more elastic and are harder to break.

	Who	What	Explanation
1.	Instructor	Claps twice	Line up (Shugo)
2.	Head student	"Ki o Tsuke"	Attention
3.	Head student	"Seiza"	Sit in kneeling position
4.	Head student	"Mokuso Hajime"	Close eyes/begin meditation
5.	Instructor	"Mokuso Yame"	Open eyes/end meditation
6.	Head student	"Dojo Kun"	Shout the Dojo Kun responsively
7.	Head student	"Shomen Ni"	Face forward (towards Shomen)
8.	Head student	"Rei"	Bow
9.	Head student	"Sensei Ni"	Face towards instructor
10.	Head student	"Rei"	Bow
11.	Everybody	"Arigato Gozaimashita"	Thank you very much for teaching me.
12.	Head student	"Yudansha Ni"	Face towards black belts or guest instructor(s)
13.	Head student	"Rei"	Bow
14.	Everybody	"Arigato Gozaimashita"	Thank you for teaching me
15.	Head student	"Otogai Ni"	Face towards other student(s)
16.	Head student	"Rei"	Bow
17.	Everybody	"Arigato Gozaimashita"	Thank you for teaching me
18.	Head student	"Shomen Ni"	Face front
19.	Instructor	"Tatsu"	Straighten or stand up
20.	Instructor	"Kurasant Jantov"	Good night (honored guests)
21.	All	Clap several times	Applause

TABLE 6. CLOSING CEREMONY

Students may then proceed to stretch their joints and then stretch their tendons, finally proceeding to build muscles, in that order. When stretching joints or tendons, it is best to work from the ground up. Muscles can only contract, so it is important to ensure students always work opposing muscle groups during strength building exercises (e.g., when doing sit-ups also do back lifts, when building biceps also work triceps).

Daruma is typically conducted with the instructor leading from the front of the class. Students perform the exercises while maintaining the same rows they lined up in at the inception of the class. To add variety and help maintain student interest, a variation may occasionally be used where the entire class is arranged in a circle. The instructor begins with an exercise then bows to the student on his or her right who leads the next exercise. In this fashion, each student has an opportunity to lead a different exercise of their choosing.

This round robin methodology works best with small classes so that time spent in *daruma* is not excessive. When the class is very large, senior students can be selected to lead portions of *daruma* as a reward for achieving rank or as practice toward when they become teachers themselves. Most children love opportunities to lead the class. Certain personality types may view public speaking associated with leading the class as a thing to be avoided at all costs, so it is advisable to ask for volunteers rather than assigning students this opportunity. (At some point it is also a good idea to encourage the more reluctant students, so that they do not miss out on this teaching experience.)

Regardless of the methods used, the purpose of *daruma* should always be to ensure that students are warmed up and ready to learn budo. It should never be conducted in such a manner that students are too exhausted to learn the martial material for which they are attending class.

My favorite technique for initiating *daruma* is the cross-march. Practitioners alternately raise their left arm/right leg, followed by their right arm/left leg to a count called by the instructor. Performed as a vigorous, in-place march, it not only provides an aerobic benefit, but helps promote cross-brain connections and reflex actions as well. A great many books and videos discuss stretching and conditioning in detail, so I'll keep the rest of this brief: In most classes I have students loosen up their ankles, knees, hips, elbows, wrists, and neck, then deeply stretch their legs, back, and wrists at minimum. Conditioning exercises generally include traditional pushups, Hindu pushups, Hindu squats, crunch sit-ups, side sit-ups, back lifts, and leg throw-downs, the latter two of which are performed with a partner. For great advice on conditioning exercises I recommend www.mattfurey.com.

For children's classes it is useful to interject unusual and interesting partner exercises such as mountain pushups, stump pushups, or dragon pushups. For mountain pushups one practitioner lies on his or her back, feet on the floor, with arms and knees held rigidly up. The other person places his or her hands on the partner's knees with legs supported by the partner over his or her head. Together they do simultaneous pushups. This requires a certain degree of strength and body control to avoid falling on each other.

For younger children, stump pushups are better and safer. Stump pushups are done with one partner being a "stump" to support the other's legs while he or she does pushups. This incline approach works the upper chest and is easier for kids to perform. Stronger kids can place just their toes on their partner's back for a tougher workout while weaker ones can support their knees there for an easier time.

Dragon pushups are a variation of this where everyone lies on the floor in a standard pushup position with their legs on someone else's back. Staggering practitioners 90 degrees to each other can connect everyone to everyone else throughout the room. The goal is for the whole class to do each repetition simultaneously so that they all push up and let down at the same time. If anyone does not pull his or her weight, the dragon collapses, so heavier/stronger students should be at one end with lighter/weaker ones at the other.

Because the upper to lower body mass ratios are higher in children, they often have difficulty performing sit-ups by themselves. A good trick is to have them face each other and lock

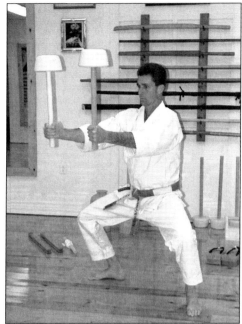

PHOTO COURTESY OF BUSHIFITNESS.COM.™

SUPPLEMENTARY TRAINING WITH VARIOUS TOOLS, *KIGU HOJO UNDO*, CAN HELP *BUDOKA* DEVEL-
OP TREMENDOUS PHYSICAL STRENGTH AND FLEXIBILITY. *CHIISHI* EXERCISES ARE DEMONSTRATED
HERE. *CHIISHI* IS A CONCRETE OR STONE WEIGHT AT THE END OF A WOODEN HANDLE USED TO
STRENGTHEN THE GRIP, AS WELL AS THE JOINTS OF THE ELBOWS, WRISTS, AND SHOULDERS.

their ankles together when doing sit-ups. If timing is reasonably
coordinated, they will be able to support each other's legs,
making a good base from which to execute the technique. They
will be able to more and better sit-ups in this fashion. Crunch
sit-ups are healthier than full sit-ups and are easier for kids to
perform correctly.

Teaching Kigu Hojo Undo
---

*"Miyagi thrust his hand into a bunch of
bamboos and pulled out one from the center.
He struck his hand into a slab of meat and tore
off chunks. He put white chalk on the bottoms
of his feet, jumped up, and kicked the ceiling—
leaving his footprints on the ceiling for all to
see. Spectators hit him with long staffs with no*

*effect. With his fingers he tore off the bark of a
tree and with his big toe he punctured a hole in
a kerosene can."* [35]

– Takuda Anshu

Hojo undo means supplemental exercises. Supplementary
training with various tools (e.g., *kigu hojo undo* or *kigu undo)*
can help *budoka* develop tremendous physical strength and
flexibility. Traditional Okinawan training equipment includes
*makiwara, ishisashi, tan, tetsuarei, chiishi, makiage kigu, nigiri
game, tou, jari bako, tetsu geta, kongoken,* and *sashi ishi.*

Much like modern free-weight equipment, the use of training apparatus greatly increases one's propensity for becoming
injured. Consequently, students must complete a thorough
warm-up prior to the commencement of *kigu hojo undo.*
Additionally, instructors should keep a watchful eye on junior
students until they have developed a sufficient level of proficiency to handle the various pieces of equipment in a controlled
and safe manner.

Makiwara is a striking post with a straw, cloth, leather, or
rubber covering for contact padding. It is used for practicing
striking techniques as well as for conditioning the hands,
elbows, knees, and feet. Younger children whose hands are still
developing should *never* punch a *makiwara.* It is too rigid and
may cause injury, so substitute a modern punching bag instead.
Ishisashi is a stone padlock resembling the shape of an old-
fashioned clothes iron. It is used for strengthening arms and
wrists. *Tan* is typically a sanded wooden log or a wooden fab-
rication resembling a barbell with weights on the ends. It is
usually rolled over the forearms or twisted over the hips to
strengthen and condition these areas. *Tetsuarei* are basic dumbbells, used much like modern weightlifting equipment.

Chiishi is a concrete or stone weight at the end of a wood-
en handle used to strengthen the grip, as well as the joints of
the elbows, wrists, and shoulders. *Chiishi* exercises condition
tendons and joints and help develop the muscles used for
blocking, striking, and grappling techniques. If the *chiishi* is
too heavy to control appropriately, practitioners should choke

up on the handle so that the weight is closer to the body. *Makiage kigu* is a wrist roller made from a wooden handle with a weight hung in the center on a rope. By twisting the handle to wrap and unwrap the rope, the weight is lowered and raised, and strengthening the forearms, wrists, and grip.

Nigiri game are gripping jars, usually made of clay with a rim around the top to grip with the fingers. Water, sand, or small stones are often added to increase the weight. Exercises with these jars are designed to strengthen the fingers for gripping and tearing applications. *Tou* is a bundle of bamboo sticks taped together at the ends. It is used for practicing finger strikes and conditioning the hands. Similarly, *jari bako*, a box or bowl filled with sand, beans, gravel or similar material, is used for finger thrusts and to toughen the hands.

Tetsu geta are iron clogs, used to strengthen kicking techniques. *Kongoken* is a very heavy rectangular hoop. Used alone or with a partner *kongoken* techniques strengthen the body and condition the *budoka* for contact. *Sashi ishi* is a short wooden handle with a stone weight in the center.

These items are traditional implements used by *Goju Ryu* practitioners as supplemental exercises. There are also modern devices that can be incorporated into training to strengthen and/or condition the body (e.g., heavy bags, speed bags, jump ropes, medicine balls, free weights, etc.).

Codification of Technique and Learning Velocity

"A kata is a pattern of movements, which contains a series of logical and practical attacking and blocking techniques... it is known that the old masters studied the combative techniques and movements in the fighting between animal and animal, animal and man, and man-to-man. They also studied the physiology of the human body and its relationship to combat, taking into account such factors as the circulation of the blood in a twenty-four hour day, the vulnerability of the vital points in relation to the time of day, and other cyclic laws of nature such as the rising and setting of the sun, and the rise and

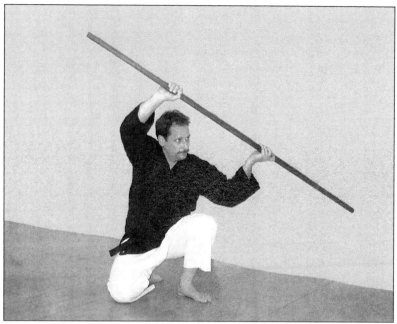

THIS IS A MOVEMENT FROM *CHUAN NO KON,* A *MATAYOSHI KOBUDO BO KATA.* A CODIFIED SYSTEM OF *KATA* FACILITATES A BUDOKA'S ABILITY TO RAPIDLY LEARN THEIR ART. IN THE UNARMED STYLES SUCH AS KARATE, *KATA* IS EVEN MORE IMPORTANT AS FAR MORE SUBTLETY IS REQUIRED TO PERFECT SUCH SKILLS.[N]

fall of the tides. All of these elements are incorporated into the kata...

"The true meaning and spirit of karate are imbedded in the kata and only by the practice of kata can we come to understand them." [36]

– Morio Higaonna Sensei, Hanshi

Historically, the major difference between European and Asian martial arts was the codification of *kata,* predefined sequences of blocks, strikes, and patterns of movement that can be practiced solo. *Kata* facilitated consistency and velocity in passing martial techniques from teachers to students and ensured that vital knowledge could survive over many genera-

111

tions. In studying a variety of martial arts over the years, I have found that I personally learn much faster when *kata* is integrated into a curriculum and believe that almost all practitioners would have similar experiences.

Information on style and technique in the Orient was historically passed on from master to student using oral tradition. Very little was written down, partially because literacy was quite rare outside the nobility and certain privileged merchant classes. These instructors embedded their unique fighting systems within their *kata*, which became fault-tolerant methods for ensuring that techniques could consistently be taught and understood over the generations. As students learned the basics and gained their instructor's confidence, they would be initiated into the secrets of his (or her) system.

In medieval recreation groups, such as the Society for Creative Anachronism (SCA) and the Realm of Chivalry (RoC), practitioners who excel in their arts eventually become knights, much as practitioners who master traditional Asian martial arts become black belts. In these organizations I learned how to fight with a variety of weapons using the traditional European martial approach, practicing basic thrusts, slashes, and parries under the tutelage of a knight. Once I understood the basics, I went to regular fight practices where I spent two to three hours sparring with fellow medieval enthusiasts several times a week.

While this approach was certainly fun, it relied on the individual instructor and the natural talent of the pupil. Practitioners learned the important nuances of techniques to varying degrees and progressed at varying speeds. Very little subtlety was formalized. There was almost no discussion, for example, of breathing, stance, balance, or footwork. Practitioners had to figure these things out for themselves.

While they lack pointy metal bits at their ends, *bo* staffs are used in a fashion that is very similar to that of a spear used by the medieval knights (who used quarterstaffs too, of course, but the SCA and RoC consider them too dangerous for use in modern full-contact tournaments, where armor does not always protect against crippling ankle and foot injuries). When

I began learning how to use the *bo* staff by studying *Matayoshi Kobudo*, I also learned the basic *hojo undo* exercises first. Shortly thereafter, however, I began to practice formal *kata*. These *kata* demonstrated logical progressions, combination techniques, stance applications, and proper footwork. Using this approach my *bo* skills developed much more rapidly than my spear skills had previously, even accounting for the affect of my earlier training.

While the subtleties of unarmed combat are simply not necessary with weapons forms, proper breathing and focus are emphasized in *kobudo* training in the same way they are taught in karate. Additionally, since *kata* can be practiced without a sparring partner, I was able to practice with the *bo* more regularly than I could with the spear. It also helped that I did not have to spend half an hour getting into and out of the protective gear each practice session, nor spend non-training time cleaning, polishing, and/or repairing my armor!

Contrasting these experiences has helped me truly understand the value of *kata* to facilitate rapid, consistent learning. If a codified system had been developed for the instruction of quarterstaff, glaive, spear, mace, maul, ax, sword, flail, or any other medieval weapon form, much of the trial and error could have been eliminated and practitioners would have been able to progress more quickly. In the unarmed arts such as karate, *kata* is even more important as far more subtlety is required to perfect such skills.

Teaching Kata

"Today's full-contact fighters throw devastating, lightning fast punches from a distance of less than two feet. Against this kind of speed, classical blocks and punches simply do not stand a chance. What amazes me is how a flaw of this magnitude—and one that is taught to thousands of unknowing students every day—still exists in what are, otherwise, extremely potent arts...

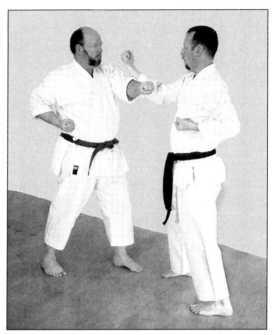

ALTHOUGH EVERYTHING HAPPENS SIMULTANEOUSLY, IT IS USEFUL TO VISUALIZE TRADITIONAL BLOCKS AS TWO-PART TECHNIQUES. IN THE FIRST MOVEMENT, THE HAND THAT IS OUT (E.G., JUST PUNCHED OR BLOCKED) INTERCEPTS THE OPPONENT'S ATTACK, RENDERING IT HARMLESS WITH A BLOCK, CHECK, OR DEFLECTION. HERE, *SENSEI* DEMONSTRATES THE FIRST MOVEMENT OF A TRADITIONAL *CHUDAN UKE* (CHEST BLOCK).°

> *"Punching with the counter hand chambered at the hip not only slows your punch (because of the distance from the target), it also creates a mammoth opening in your defense... Like the punching method, the classical blocking method—with the counter hand chambered at the hip and far from the action—takes much too long to come into play... a wind-up precedes the actual block..."*[37]
>
> – Name Withheld

Kata can be an extremely powerful, fault tolerant tool for transferring martial knowledge between teacher and student. If taught incorrectly, however, it can be used as an excuse to misinterpret or bastardize an otherwise effective martial art.

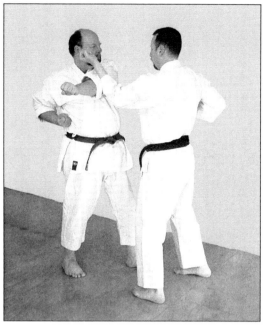

ONCE THE ATTACK HAS BEEN NEUTRALIZED VIA A BLOCK, CHECK, OR DEFLECTION FROM THE FORWARD ARM, *KARATEKA* SEIZE ADVANTAGE, CONTROLLING THEIR OPPONENT USING THE OTHER (CHAMBERED) HAND. BLOCKS TO THE OUTSIDE ARE DONE ABOVE THE ELBOW TO CLOSE WITH AN OPPONENT. WHILE AN ATTACKER MAY ONLY BE CROSSED-UP FOR AN INSTANT, THIS ENTANGLEMENT GIVES THE PRACTITIONER ENOUGH TIME FOR AT LEAST ONE COUNTER-ATTACK.[P]

According to Morio Higaonna *Sensei*, the true meaning and the spirit of karate are imbedded in *kata*. Only through the practice of *kata* can we come to understand them. For this reason, if we were to change or simplify *kata*, either to accommodate beginners or for tournament purposes, then we would also lose the true meaning and the spirit of karate.

While multiple interpretations of each movement within a *kata* are possible (see *Teaching Bunkai*), all practitioners should execute the movements of each *kata* in exactly the same way every time. In this fashion the core foundation of the art is preserved. Once practitioners understand the gross movements of a new *kata*, it is essential for instructors to delve into subtleties in a manner appropriate to each student.

Instructors should teach adults a little more than they can remember such that more and more knowledge is internalized each time. Children, on the other hand, should be taught in smaller bites. Either way, only the newest of the new students might misinterpret fundamental truisms such as the "wind-up" misconception quoted above.

Dispelling the "Wind-up" Block Misconception

The quote at the beginning of this section represents a fundamental flaw—both in the teaching of *kata,* and understanding thereof, by the individual quoted. The point of including this quotation is not to disparage its author, however. Such misjudgments are quite common and reflect more on poor teaching than on anything else. Contrary to this misperception, the hand that is out (e.g., just punched or blocked) performs the actual block, check, or deflection, while the hand that is in chamber executes a technique designed to control the opponent's limb. Even though it is often hidden, almost all blocks in *Goju Ryu kata* utilize this check/control methodology.

Most "traditional" karate forms, in fact, utilize this approach. In all cases, there is never any "wind-up" preceding anything. Common misconceptions such as this one are the reason that I believe it is imperative to supplement the traditional modeling approach to martial arts instruction with lecturing, cooperative performance, and other teaching styles.

To delve deeper, the word *"uke"* translates more accurately to "receive" than it does to "block." When viewed in this context, it may be easier to understand that practitioners typically check, deflect, or control an attack rather than meeting it force-on-force. Using the traditional check/control methodology, a practitioner's outstretched hand need only deflect an attack by a few inches to spoil its effect when contact is made close to an opponent's body.

In this fashion *karateka* can easily avoid being hit by even the most "devastating" of punches no matter how fast, or how powerfully, or even how unexpectedly they are thrown. Blocks to the outside are done above the elbow to close with an opponent and avoid follow-on elbow strikes, while blocks to the inside are done below the elbow to open an opponent and avoid subsequent follow-through or whipping blows.

When done properly, blocks will always feel like attacks to an opponent. In fact, I have seen more than one case of someone either hyper-extending or breaking an attacker's arm while blocking his punch during a real fight.

Debunking the "Ineffectual" Punch Myth

Fighting ranges in *Goju Ryu* karate are extremely close. Classical punches in our style, as with most traditional karate forms, are done such that as one hand moves out toward the opponent the other moves back into chamber at the practitioner's side. As the aforementioned quote indicates, this has been perceived as being too slow to do any good in a real fight. In reality, however, this *hikite* (push/pull) technique aligns the *karateka*'s body in a manner that facilitates speed and power in their attack. Through proper body alignment, the practitioner's weight and the force of gravity are added to the punch making it massively more effective than a reliance on muscular strength alone.

Goju Ryu translates as "hard, soft style," with *go* meaning "hard" and *ju* meaning "soft" or "gentle." Punches (and kicks for that matter) in *Goju Ryu* are executed while the practitioner's muscles are loose to achieve maximum speed. *Karateka* then tense their entire bodies, contracting their muscles at the precise moment of impact to ensure crisp, solid blows. Similar to cracking a whip, this facilitates great quickness and power.

Using this technique, masters of classical Okinawan karate can kill someone with a single blow (though incidents of that happening are rare). I get bruises every time I practice with a *Naha-Te* (an indigenous Okinawan form of karate) black belt who is nearly twice my age. He is no longer as physically strong as he once was, but his body alignment is perfect, and he uses his mastery of internal power to throw me around the *dojo* with ease.

Even if one is not a master, however, there is more than one type of punch in karate, and more than one vector from which it can be thrown. Jabs, uppercuts, swing strikes, knife-hand strikes, and a multitude of other techniques abound. Several hand configurations are used as well, including the traditional horizontal fist, vertical (standing) fist, one-knuckle punch, palm heel strike, and finger thrust. In any given tactical situation, practitioners will select their most effective attack, optimizing angle, distance, timing, and hand position. This much is fairly obvious in most *kata*.

What is hidden to the casual observer is that the hand returning to chamber quite often has something in it, indicating a pull or a grab. In this fashion most attacks unbalance an opponent while causing simultaneous physiological damage, a highly potent combination. When this grab and strike cross the centerline of an opponent's body, the potential for neurological damage is increased as well. Pressure point/nerve strikes take advantage of this. When properly applied, *kata* fundamentals make classical karate punches (as well as blocks and kicks) highly effective, indeed devastatingly so.

A Three Step Approach to Learning *Kata*

I have found that the vast majority of practitioners learn new *kata* most efficiently using a three-step approach, as follows:

- Do the *kata* as many times as it takes to understand the basic pattern.
- Explore the *kata bunkai* to recognize some possible interpretations of the various applications contained therein (see *Teaching Bunkai* below).
- Repeat the *kata* several more times, keeping the *bunkai* in mind.

A *kata* is never really learned until its *bunkai* are thoroughly understood. Once the basics of a new *kata* have been internalized, students can progress toward learning the more esoteric components such as nerve strikes, angles of attack, and hidden applications.

Beginning and Ending a Kata

To begin a *kata*, a karate practitioner stands in *masubi dachi* (attention stance) with both hands at the sides and bows. The practitioner says aloud the name of the *kata* he or she will be demonstrating, then lifts both hands together (left over right with palms towards the body) up to chest height in front then down to *yoi* (ready position) at the waist keeping the left hand over the right (palms toward the body). This is actually part of the *kata* so it needs to be done with focus and vigor. From there the practitioner may begin or may step into the first stance of the *kata* in a *kamae* (combative posture) position and then begin.

To end a *kata* after completing all the movements, a practitioner once again stands in *masubi dachi* with both hands at the sides and bows. If you are in a line with other students and have not returned to the *kiten* point (the physical point in the room from which the *kata* was initiated), you may be required to follow-up with a *yanjigo* (diagonal step) to re-center yourself (along with everyone else) in the room. While the *yanjigo* is not part of the actual *kata* itself, without this movement practitioners would eventually shift off the training floor.

Although some variation in curricula exists, the core *katas* of *Goju Ryu* karate typically include, *gekisai* (*dai ichi* and *dai ni*), *saifa, seiyunchin, seisan, saipai, shisochin, sanseiru, kurunfa, sanchin, tensho,* and *suparinpei.* Many schools begin with *taikyoku* (*gedan, chudan,* and *jodan*) and/or *hookiyu kata.* Some schools also teach *gekiha (dai ichi* and *dai ni*), and/or *kakuha.* Each martial system, be it judo, karate, aikido, kung fu, tai chi, kendo, or any other codified art form will have a core curricula similar to this one. Every Asian martial art that I have studied utilizes *kata* at the heart of its system. Emphasis, strategy, and techniques vary, of course, but the concept remains the same. For more detailed information about the *katas* of *Goju Ryu* karate, see appendix B (*Kata of Goju Ryu*).

Teaching Bunkai

"It should be known that the secret principles of Goju Ryu karate exist in the kata." [38]

– *Chojun Miyagi Sensei*

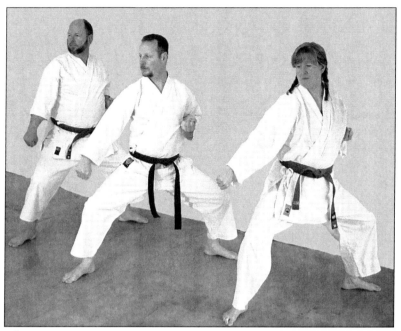

ACCORDING TO THE SECOND RULE OF *KAISAI*, WHAT APPEARS TO BE FORWARD MOVING DOWN BLOCKS IN SEIYUNCHIN *KATA*, MUST REALLY BE ATTACKS. ALTHOUGH THE MOVEMENTS ARE ALWAYS DONE IN THE SAME MANNER, KEEPING APPLICATIONS IN MIND WILL STRENGTHEN THE EXECUTION OF ONE'S *KATA*.[Q]

Bunkai are applications or fighting techniques found in *kata*. When executing the *kata*, however, such movements are typically stylized with their actual applications obscured. Although a formal set of applications, or *kata bunkai oyo*, have been developed for most *katas*, nearly limitless interpretations may apply.

While *kata* are always done exactly the same way, *kata bunkai* allow for more spontaneity and experimentation within a standard framework. In *kata bunkai* practitioners use techniques in prearranged manners with a partner to better understand the emphasis and meaning of the various *katas* that they have learned. Almost all *katas* in *Goju Ryu* have predefined *bunkai* associated with them.

These standard sequences, however, are only the beginning. There are numerous "correct" interpretations for each movement of every *kata*, each demonstrating a functional, real-life application.

The work to uncover hidden techniques in *kata* is called *kaisai*. Since it offers guidelines for unlocking the secrets of each *kata, kaisai no genri* (the Theory of *Kaisai*) was once a great mystery revealed only to trusted disciples of the ancient masters in order to protect the secrets of their system.

While a large number of rules exist, the three main principles of *Kaisai No Genri* are as follows:

1. Do not be deceived by the *enbusen* rule.
2. Techniques executed while advancing imply attacking techniques while those executed while retreating imply defensive or blocking techniques.
3. There is only one enemy and he or she is in front of you.

Enbusen literally means "lines for performance" of fighting techniques. *Kata* are choreographed using artificial symmetry to ensure that the practitioner never takes more than three or four steps in any one direction, a process of conserving required practice space. These short movements obviously have nothing to do with real fighting situations. Similarly, punching left does not necessarily mean that you fight against an enemy on your left side.

Kata technique executed while advancing should be considered an attack, even if it appears to be defensive. Similarly, those techniques executed while retreating should imply defensive or blocking techniques, even if they look like attacks. For example, in *seiyunchin kata*, there are many *gedan uke* (low blocks) executed while moving forward in *shiko dachi* (sumo or straddle stance). It seems somewhat odd to be blocking while moving forward, especially in this low stance. According to the second rule of *kaisai*, these must be offensive rather than defensive techniques. Using this rule, *kata* applications become usable in real life situations.

As *karateka* face toward many directions moving along lines of *enbusen*, they might believe that *kata* were created to emulate situations wherein one person fights against several opponents at the same time. The origin of *kata*, however, was in two-man tandem sparring. Consequently, the *kumite* are

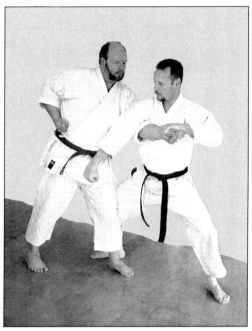

ONE INTERPRETATION OF THE DOWN BLOCK FROM SEIYUNCHIN *KATA* IS THAT YOU HAVE CAP-
TURED AN OPPONENT'S ARM AND ARE MOVING IN FOR A DOWNWARD STRIKE TO THE GROIN, A
POWERFUL PUSH-PULL TECHNIQUE. LOW STANCES SUCH AS *SHIKO DACHI* ARE EXECUTED VERY
CLOSE TO AN OPPONENT AND CAN BE USED TO CRASH THROUGH AND UPROOT BALANCE TO
SUPPLEMENT AN ATTACK.[R]

also one-on-one. These dance-like direction shifts were created
to keep the movement concise, not to imply multiple attackers.

In reality, from a street-fighting point of view, it is pretty
much impossible to make a *kata* that is designed to fight
against multiple attackers at once. One person cannot simultaneously execute many different techniques against multiple
opponents except in well-choreographed movie stunts.
Although there are some *kata* where the imaginary enemy
strikes from behind, there is always only one opponent at a
time. Once the first opponent has been defeated, a *karateka* can
move on to defeat the next attacker (multiple attackers are generally handled by strategically engaging one at a time in a manner that confounds the others ability to reach you).

Using the three main principles of *kaisai no genri* practitioners can decipher the original intent of *kata* techniques by

logically analyzing each specific technique to find its hidden meaning. After finding what one believes is the application of a *kata* technique, it must be examined to determine whether or not it would be effective in actual combat. To do this *karateka* can practice the technique in a *kumite* (sparring) situation with a partner; in essence reverse engineering the original *kata*. This is how many of the original *kiso kumites* (prearranged sparring drills) were developed.

It is a good idea to devote time on a regular basis to practice and discuss the principles of *kaisai no genri* with senior students. In this manner they gain practical understanding of the main principles above, and they also can develop and test their own theories, defining corollary principles in a meaningful and personal way. This goes a long way toward strengthening their abilities to apply concepts found in the various *kata* that they practice to real life situations.

Once corollary principle, for example, states that where you touch your own body in *kata* indicates where to strike on the opponent. Using this theory, one finds not only direct, obvious applications, but obscure, subtle ones as well: In *saipai kata, bensoku dachi* (crossed-foot stance, a somewhat awkward transitional movement), might demonstrate entangling an opponent's legs causing disruption that can be exploited with the follow-up *furi uchi* (swing strike).

Another corollary principle is that a hand in chamber (held by your side) usually has something in it, indicating a grab or pull. Combining this with the second rule of *kaisai* above gives greater meaning to the forward moving down blocks in *seiyunchin kata*. Clearly one interpretation is that you have captured an opponents arm and are moving in for a downward strike to the groin, a powerful push-pull technique.

Since *shiko dachi* (sumo stance) is a powerful low stance, you are probably crashing through and uprooting their balance as well. And if you add the ear slap that typically precedes a down block (another corollary principle—strike to disrupt; disrupt to strike), this becomes an even more effective application as another layer of disruption precedes the groin strike.

Clearly, there is a lot more going on in *kata* than is readily

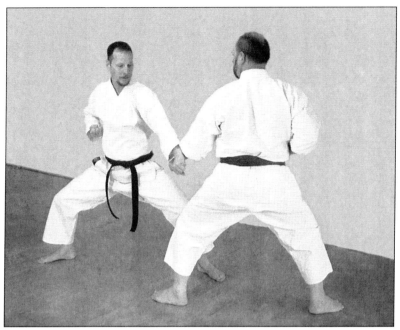

WHEN TEACHING *KUMITE* TO NEW STUDENTS, IT IS A GOOD IDEA TO START SLIGHTLY OUT OF RANGE SUCH THAT ACCIDENTS ARE LESS LIKELY TO OCCUR. *SENSEI* DEMONSTRATES ONE INTERPRETATION OF THE DOWN BLOCK FROM *SEIYUNCHIN KATA*. SINCE THIS IS DONE OUT OF RANGE AND TREATED MERELY AS A BLOCK, THE OPPONENT IS FREE TO CONTINUE ATTACKING. THIS APPROACH MAKES A DECENT MOVING DRILL BUT IS NOT A VERY EFFECTIVE IN ACTUAL COMBAT. EVEN THOUGH NEWER STUDENTS WILL NOT PRACTICE IN FIGHTING RANGE FOR SAFETY REASONS, THEY MUST UNDERSTAND WHAT IS USEFUL IN REAL LIFE AND WHAT IS NOT.[5]

apparent to the untrained observer. Without practical applications, students might as well be Jazzercising™. Teaching *bunkai* is a powerful method for imparting essential martial knowledge to karate students. Similar principles are utilized in other martial art forms as well.

Teaching Kiso Kumite

"Kumite is the creative process by which one applies everything learned in basics and kata and uses it while under the pressure of combat." [39]

– Dr. George W. Alexander Sensei, Kudan

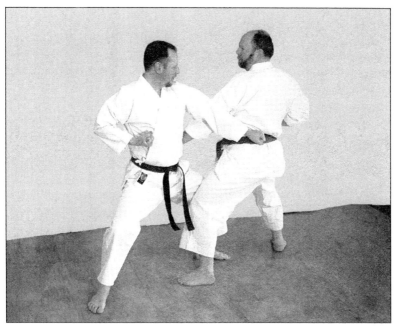

SENSEI DEMONSTRATES A MORE REALISTIC INTERPRETATION OF THE DOWN BLOCK FROM *SEIYUNCHIN KATA*. SINCE IT IS TREATED AS AN ATTACK THIS TIME, THE OPPONENT CAN BE DISABLED. NOTE THAT THE ELBOW AND KIDNEYS ARE STRUCK SIMULTANEOUSLY. (THIS MOVE-MENT ACTUALLY BEGINS WITH DEFLECTION FROM THE RIGHT HAND IMMEDIATELY FOLLOWED BY AN EAR SLAP FROM THE LEFT TO DISRUPT THE ATTACKER. IN ONE CONTINUOUS MOTION THE LEFT HAND CROSSES OVER THE OPPONENT'S HEAD AND DRIVES DOWN INTO THE ELBOW/KIDNEY STRIKE). WHEN SHOWN AT PROPER FIGHTING DISTANCE, THIS BECOMES A SUBSTANTIALLY MORE EFFECTIVE TECHNIQUE.[T]

Kiso Kumite is a set of attack and counter attack sequences designed to teach self-defense skills without the dangers inherent in free sparring. Techniques are pulled from a variety of *katas* and grouped by theme (e.g., evasion, nerve strikes, short techniques, elbows strikes). *Ippon kumite* uses only the last attack and defense from each set, followed by an additional set of freeform attacks by the original defender.

As *kata* are always done exactly the same way and *kata bunkai* allow for more spontaneity, *kiso kumite* allows for an even wider range of experimentation to really define what works for each individual practitioner while keeping to a standard framework. *Goshin do ippon kumite* affords students the opportunity to make up their own self-defense sequences based

> katas they are studying.

When teaching *kumite* to new students, it is a good idea to start slightly out of range such that accidents are less likely to occur. Once students are somewhat familiar with techniques and have achieved an appropriate level of control, applications can be performed within contact range. Junior students always initiate attacks, while senior students defend. In this manner, the junior students always know what to expect and are able to emulate what they have seen. The attacker typically makes a long first step, while the defender makes a shorter one to execute techniques in the proper range.

Once students understand the movements and have enough control to complete techniques safely, they should begin to practice in actual fighting ranges. It is important that they be taught to give pressure and to honor their partner's techniques. Giving pressure means using proper body alignment and good stances such that forward pressure against the opponent is maintained at all times. This approximates realistic conditions where only well-executed movements will be effective. Honoring technique means reacting as if one has been struck with significant force such that practitioners can practice combinations of technique in a realistic manner.

Teaching Self-Defense

"Street fighting is not martial arts. It is between you and an enemy, who is trying to injure, maim, rape, or kill you. Whoever is attacking you has probably done it before and more than likely enjoys it. He has probably been hit hard before and has learned how to shrug off pain. You need to hurt him in a way that impairs his body's ability to function and takes him out of the fight." [40]

– *Massad Ayoob,*
Director of the Lethal Force Institute

As previously mentioned, *kata* are always done exactly the same way, and *bunkai* and *kumite* allow for more flexibility and experimentation within a prescribed framework. However, all bets are off when it comes to real life self-defense. Self-defense techniques are a foundation on which to build creativity, spontaneity, and to define multiple applications from any given technique. Size mismatches, unexpected actions by opponents, and other variables need to be considered and compensated for.

Students must understand that there is no "magic bullet" technique to fit all situations. In short, once a confrontation begins, practitioners must do whatever works to end it quickly. A fundamental principle of karate, however, is that all techniques should be applied defensively. Martial artists should never *provoke* confrontations. While there certainly are situations in which fighting is the only alternative, it is best to avoid physical altercations altogether whenever possible.

Avoiding Violence

> *"People should learn to see and so avoid all danger. Just as a wise man keeps away from mad dogs, so one should not make friends with evil men."* [41]
>
> *– Buddha*

The only way to guarantee victory in a physical confrontation is to walk away before the first blow is thrown. Although martial artists train to survive (or even triumph) in a fight, students should be taught to do everything they can to *avoid* violence in the first place. They can use humor, deception, bribery, or any other plausible tactic that might work. Even if a person legitimately uses force in order to escape imminent and unavoidable danger, they still have to live with the physiological, psychological, and legal results of doing so.

Martial artists frequently develop a feeling of invulnerability and begin to court danger in ways they never would have prior to beginning their training. Sauntering through a dark alley in a bad neighborhood after midnight, leering at a professional ballplayer's girlfriend at a nightclub, and antagonizing protesters at a political rally are all bad ideas no matter how well trained (or armed) you happen to be. Students should understand that the more dangerous they are, the less they should feel a need to prove it. It is far better to withdraw than it is to face the consequences of causing or allowing an argument to escalate to the point of physical confrontation.

When I was twelve years old, I was walking to the bus stop after judo practice one night when four older boys stopped me. They quickly began to hassle me about the *gi* I was wearing, spitting on me, calling me names, and threatening to "kill" me. Verbal threats soon escalated to pushing and shoving, which was clearly evolving toward more serious blows. Although I probably stood a good chance of badly injuring one or two of them, I felt that there was no way I could win a fight against four kids, all of whom were bigger, older, and most likely stronger than I was.

Swallowing my pride, I did my best to ignore their expectorating and taunting while I tried to figure out a way to escape. As soon as I saw a car approaching, I shoved the nearest antagonist out of the way, shoulder-rolled over the hood of the vehicle, and darted across the street. The driver slammed on his brakes, stopping between where I had just run and where the bullies on sidewalk had started to follow. While they were distracted by the irate driver, I hopped over a fence, ducked down another side street, and ran away as fast as I could. In a situation where I could not win, running was clearly the best thing to do.

A dozen years later, I was accosted in the Pioneer Square area of Seattle (Washington) by two street thugs who demanded that I give them money. Both had large belt knives clearly visible, but not yet drawn. Both were large, muscular, and outweighed me by more than forty pounds each. If it came to a fight this time, however, there was no way that the bad guys could win.

Although they did not know it, these muggers were not the only ones who were armed. I have a concealed pistol license and was carrying a gun hidden beneath my jacket.[42] Once again, I had to make a choice between swallowing my pride and handing over some money or escalating a conflict toward an undoubtedly lethal ending.

Legally I had a pretty good case for forcefully defending myself, as I was confronted by two larger, obviously armed individuals and in reasonable fear for my life. Morally and ethically, however, I knew that there was a better choice. Pulling a small wad of bills from my pocket, I threw the money to one side then immediately ran to the other.[43]

Had these thugs decided to chase me, I would most likely have had no choice but to meet their attack with countervailing force. Fortunately, however, they took long enough picking-up the $27.00 I had left behind that I got away. I consider that a small price to pay to avoid having to kill or maim two people, even if they clearly were bad guys.

For children who are physically weaker and emotionally less resilient than adults, avoiding violence is especially important. They should be taught to use their feet rather than their martial skills to escape conflict. Let's face it, no matter how well trained an 80-pound child might be, he or she will have little chance of success against a 280-pound, hardened criminal. Using one's wits becomes extremely important. A child yelling for help, for example, will receive less attention from bystanders than one that yells, "That's not my dad!" or "Help, that's not my dad!"

I believe that it is imperative to teach students that while conflict cannot always be avoided, it is always prudent to try. When confrontation becomes inevitable, however, a proper mind-set will help them survive.

Self-Defense Mind Set

> *"Everyone has a plan; then they get punched in the mouth."* [44]

> – *"Iron" Mike Tyson,*
> *former world heavyweight*
> *boxing champion*

all the techniques necessary to defend oneself in a ... ure fight are found in *kata, kata bunkai,* and *kiso kumite,* the most important thing to emphasize when teaching self-defense to *karate* students is mind-set. Street fighting is not about winning. It is about *not* losing!

According to Massad Ayoob, a seasoned street fighter will usually beat a karate expert who has never been in a real fight. In order to survive, a practitioner must be prepared to ignore the pain while mercilessly counterattacking their assailant. Remember, if it hurts, you are still alive.

In a real fight, martial arts training can take over automatically. *Budoka* can literally watch their bodies perform what they have been trained to do, with fists and feet or makeshift weapons, without having to think about it all that much. That is why students are taught to practice repetitively and realistically. When real danger arises, pre-programmed responses can take over.

Instructors should encourage students to apply techniques from training that fit personality, physique, and general physical condition. Students should focus on being offensive. They should not try to get fancy, but simply think "him, down, now." Utilize vital area attacks whenever possible to enhance the chances of success. In order to deliver blows with maximum force, practitioners should aim their attacks through opponents, rather than at him/her.

Real fighting is nothing like training in the *dojo.* There are no rules in a real fight. Students should be instructed not to believe anything an attacker says. They should do anything to survive. A practitioner should not stop until the attacker has been disabled and/or the practitioner can safely get away.

Once a real-life confrontation escalates into combat, adrenaline rushes through a person's system. This dramatically increases pain tolerance and helps a person survive in fighting mode. This "fight or flight" reaction instantly supercharges the body for a short period of time, increasing pulse rate and blood pressure, while making a person faster, meaner, and more impervious to pain than ever before. Teach your students to embrace their fear in a fight; it can help them survive.

Moral and Legal Aspects

"You may find yourself tangling with criminals or terrorists. Sometimes you'll need to neutralize them until the police arrive, and sometimes you'll be forced to kill. Either way you must act on moral, ethical, and legal principles that are based totally on the circumstances. ...Use discretion. Remember that you're the good guy and act like one."

– W. Hock Hochheim Sensei,
Black Belt Hall of Fame member

It is imperative, however, to teach more than just avoidance, more than just technique, and more than just mind-set when discussing self-defense. Moral and legal implications absolutely, positively must be stressed as well. Martial artists learn a plethora of potentially deadly techniques and must exercise proper judgment regarding when, if, and how to use them (as I believe I demonstrated in my close encounters with violence described previously).

I am a martial artist not an attorney, therefore nothing in this document constitutes a legal opinion nor should any of its contents be treated as such. Having said that, however, the classic rule is that self-defense begins when deadly danger begins, ends when the danger ends, and revives again if the danger returns. Neither a killing that takes place after a crime has already been committed, nor a proactive violent defense before an attack has taken place is legitimate self-defense.

A person can only resort to deadly force in order to escape imminent and unavoidable danger of death or grave bodily harm. An attacker must not merely have made a threat to attack someone, but must be in a position where he or she is obviously and immediately capable of carrying out that threat and/or has begun to do so. In one case my attackers threatened to kill me but did not demonstrate any actual intention of doing so. In the other, they clearly had the ability to kill me but had not yet initiated an attack.

A cornerstone of a legitimate claim of self-defense is the innocence of the claimant. A person must be entirely without fault. If a student begins a conflict, he or she cannot claim self-defense. If the student allows a conflict to escalate into a lethal situation when it could have been avoided, he or she shares some degree of culpability and, once again, cannot claim self-defense.

This cannot be overemphasized. There are countless stories of martial artists picking fights they regret for the rest of their lives because people were maimed or killed and the practitioners are subsequently sued or jailed or both.

Depending on the circumstances, almost any form of physical assault can be considered deadly force, which is defined in Washington State as, *"the intentional application of force through the use of firearms or any other means reasonably likely to cause death or serious physical injury."*[46] Any blow delivered powerfully and deliberately to a vital part of the body may be construed as deadly force so long as it can be shown that it was struck with the intention, or predictable likelihood, of killing.

The courts are more likely to interpret such as blow as deadly force if the person delivering it is

- physically much stronger than the victim,
- a professional fighter,
- a trained martial artist, or
- an assailant who attacks with extreme savagery.

An example of "extreme savagery" would be gratuitously raining blows upon a fallen opponent or one who has obviously given up a conflict, even if he or she started the fight. While a great majority of deadly force cases involve the use of weapons, martial arts students stand a good chance of being charged with a crime resulting from an unarmed confrontation if they are arrested and their training background is uncovered.

Equal force doctrines require law-abiding citizens to respond to an attack with little or no more force than that which he or she perceives is being directed against him or her.

Disparity of force between unarmed combatants is measured in one of two ways: it exists if the victim is being attacked by someone who is physically much stronger or bigger than he or she, or by two or more attackers of similar or equal size.

Nowhere can a person legally respond to an assault of slight degree with deadly force. In some places, the law clearly specifies that equal force must be exactly that: the attacked can respond with no more force than that by which he or she is threatened—slap for slap, kick for kick, or deadly weapon for deadly weapon.

Practically, students will usually want to respond to an assault with a degree of force sufficiently, but not greatly, superior to that with which they were threatened. There are two advantages to a "slightly greater" degree of force doctrine:

- It places the defender in a more secure tactical position.
- It discourages the assailant from continuing his or her attack and escalating into a situation where lethal force is warranted.

A great majority of states require that citizens avoid a conflict whenever possible. It is best to withdraw, leaving the scene entirely. At the very least, people are expected to retreat from a belligerent party who threatens them; unless the attack is so savage that there is no time to escape or if turning your back (or leaving cover during a gunfight) to escape would increase your vulnerability. The only exception to this rule is within the confines of a person's own home (and in some places one's business). In most cases, if someone breaks into a person's home and assaults him or her, the homeowner does not legally need to attempt to retreat (although in some cases it may be prudent to do so anyway).

Tell your students that if they are cornered and have to fight, they must also be in reasonable fear for their lives prior to applying countervailing force. For example, if an armed assailant threatens them, they should shout something like, "Oh my god, don't kill me with that knife!" Not only may this

133

attract the attention of a possible rescuer, but it also demonstrates for potential witnesses that they are, indeed, in reasonable fear for their lives.

Summary

By following a structure of merit, such as the belt system, instructors can monitor the development and skill progression of their students and can teach them according to set standards. Training objectives must be stated in terms specific enough that students will know whether or not they have been accomplished. Continuous feedback is essential in order to assure that students may understand how they are progressing. In this fashion, they are able to identify deficient areas upon which they should focus their training. Instructors should monitor student performance over time and promote them once they have met predefined proficiency levels.

Lessons should be approached within a "Plan–Do–Check–Act" framework, allowing for optimal utilization of teacher/student interaction and classroom time management. Under this process, midcourse corrections will ensure that progress is continually achieved and lessons are effectively communicated to the entire student population.

Classes should progress through a logical order that both assists in communication and facilitates efficient use of available time. Each training session should begin and end with a short ceremony to show respect for the head instructor, guest instructors, the *dojo*, and fellow students. This helps differentiate *budo* training from mundane activities, reinforces essential traditions, demonstrates proper etiquette, and gets students ready to learn.

Most classes will incorporate elements of *daruma*, *kigu undo*, *kata*, *bunkai*, *kiso kumite*, and/or self-defense applications. *Daruma* provides a proper warm-up to prevent injuries and energize students for *budo* instruction. Supplementary training with *kigu hojo undo* equipment can help students develop needed strength and flexibility. Neither activity should be conducted in such a manner that students are too exhausted to learn the martial material for which they are attending class.

Kata is the core foundation of most martial arts. The theory of *kaisai no genri* allows *karateka* to ascertain practical applications, or *bunkai*, from the *kata* they practice. *Kiso kumite*, or tandem sparring drills, facilitates practice of these techniques without the dangers inherent in free sparring where joint manipulation, vital point attacks, and nerve techniques could cause serious injury or death. It is important to give pressure and to honor a partner's techniques so that only realistic applications will be successful.

Although *kata* are always done exactly the same way, and *bunkai* and *kumite* allow for more flexibility and experimentation within a prescribed framework, all bets are off when it comes to real life self-defense. Self-defense techniques are a foundation on which to build creativity, spontaneity, and to define multiple applications from any given technique. Such instruction would be negligent, however, if it does not incorporate a comprehensive understanding of the moral and legal aspects of self-defense.

There is no first strike in karate. Martial artists should never provoke confrontations. While there certainly are situations in which fighting is the only alternative, it is best to avoid physical altercations altogether whenever possible. Once a confrontation begins, however, *budoka* must do whatever it takes to end it quickly.

CHAPTER 6

❋ Conclusion ❋

"Truth of the matter is I learn everywhere I go. I have a HUGE library of books and courses on health and fitness. Even the things that I think I already know have levels upon levels of depth. Each day as I train, I come up with variations of what I already think I know. Fact is, I'm learning what I 'thought' I knew better and better all the time."[47]

– Matt Furey

This book has covered quite a bit of material, holistically addressing martial arts instruction from a variety of interconnected directions. The first two chapters discussed learning styles and personality types to give educators a better understanding of the students they teach. The third chapter demonstrated how and when to apply each of the six primary teaching styles to martial arts. Chapter 4 addressed how to foster a positive learning environment, advocating the importance of etiquette and tradition in martial arts as well as giving special attention to the characteristics of exemplary students and exemplary instructors. Chapter 5 addressed discrete elements of lesson planning for the *dojo* and is backed up by appendix D, which contains a completed lesson plan example.

In reviewing this material, readers will probably categorize themselves as either instructors or as students, but in reality the vast majority of us fall into both categories. Although I teach a couple of karate classes every week, I take formal lessons from my instructors too. As the quote at the beginning of this chapter indicates, the more often someone practices a technique, the greater the likelyhood that he or she is likely to discover a nuance or perspective that might have been previously missed. In this way both the teacher and student roles are experienced. Furthermore, when students are actively engaged in the learning process, they frequently take on a teaching role, even if only for a small portion of the class or during extra practice with peers between formal sessions. I believe it is useful to view these materials through both the lens of the student and the teacher.

The last chapter of this book reviews the growth and progression of teaching skills and how they change over time.

Stages of Teaching

"Self understanding is the key to becoming a great teacher." [48]

– Ed Wells

New teachers pass through three relatively distinct developmental phases: induction, consolidation, and mastery. For full-time educators, the first stage typically takes about a year, while the second may take as many as five to eight years. Just as it is essential to understand the personality types and learning styles of one's students, it is also important to understand the natural progression that teachers follow throughout their careers.

Induction Stage

During the induction period, teachers begin to understand how to assess student personalities and style predilections, how to match teaching styles with lesson plans, and how to develop content to most effectively deliver essential curricula components. They learn the basics of motivating and providing feedback to students along with classroom management and discipline. It is an awkward time where theory meets reality and new teachers must assess their own strengths and weaknesses. As I personally discovered, even if one has taught before in some other capacity it takes a while to translate skills associated with teaching academic subjects to those required for teaching physical activities.

Consolidation Stage

In consolidation, teachers refine their understanding to deliver developmentally appropriate lessons, more effectively tailoring materials to individual students. Observational skills are sharpened and the "Plan–Do–Check–Act" cycle requires less conscious effort. Switching between teaching styles also becomes an instinctive process, enhancing class flow and content delivery. It is a time of progress where weaknesses are shored-up, and strengths are enhanced.

Mastery Stage

Mastery is evolutionary and may take a lifetime to truly achieve. On the journey toward mastery, teachers learn through experience and hard work to develop lessons that are enjoyable and beneficial, effective and satisfying for all involved. Delivery seems effortless as most challenges have been encountered and overcome many times before. People are not born master teachers any more than they are born master martial artists. Although they may have many of the characteristics for success at teaching, it is only through experience and continuing effort that they are able to truly master the art of education.

Conclusion

"A black belt, even a first degree black belt, must possess more than technical proficiency. He must also possess a maturity greatly exceeding his skill. A black belt must also have an understanding of the principles employed in his art and be able to pass that knowledge, skill, leadership, and maturity on to others in a precise, clear, and systemic manner. All these things are what makes a 'black belt,' a black belt." [49]

– Bob Orlando Sensei

To paraphrase Dr. Sang Kim, innate teaching methods are largely determined by an instructor's character, cultural-heritage, personality, and martial arts background. This means that there can be as many different teaching methods as there are teachers. Regardless, there are fundamental formulas that can be applied to anyone's teaching style to make it as effective as possible.

The instructor's attitude is paramount to effective communication. Martial arts are competency-based, not letter-graded along a curve. When instructors believe that their primary role is to impart knowledge, they will creatively find appropriate mechanisms to ensure that their students learn. We cannot bemoan, belittle, become irritated about, or ignore our students' legitimate needs to learn. We must exercise patience until we find effective ways of communicating to each one of them directly.

Instructors must utilize a variety of teaching styles to ensure effective communication, matching the styles to the appropriate situations. Addressing individual learning styles to the extent possible is critical to the success of class participants. Since different people learn in different ways, it is important that educators avoid the common trap of treating others as though they had the same characteristics and preferences as the instructor.

Martial arts instructors must strive to go beyond merely communicating techniques to their students, however. Consciously or unconsciously, martial artists are in unique positions to serve as role models for their students whether they intend to or not. Consequently, etiquette and tradition become essential aspects of martial arts training, for without them we would practice nothing more than base violence.

An essential tradition in karate (as with many martial arts) is that practitioners, regardless of rank, bow to each other before practicing together saying, "*Dozo one gaishimasu*" which means, "Please teach me." The implication of this tradition is that teachers can learn from their students as much as students can learn from their instructors.

In his famous book *Zen in the Martial Arts* Joe Hyams

Sensei described his first encounter with Ed Parker, the founder of American Kenpo Karate. Parker *Sensei* told him, "I am not going to show you my art. I am going to share it with you. If I show it to you it becomes an exhibition, and in time it will be pushed so far into the back of your mind that it will be lost. But by sharing it with you, you will not only retain it forever, but I, too, will improve."[50]

By preparing themselves to teach others, *budoka* gain a greater depth of understanding and further the development of themselves and their art. Teaching is not only a noble profession, but also one that is essential to truly mastering any martial art.

Hokusei Yudanshakai Advancement Requirements
☀ (through Shodan) ☀

The following is a complete listing of all advancement requirements through the rank of *shodan*. As such, this listing represents the vast majority of the curricula of this system (the remaining *katas* (*kururunfa*, *sanseiru*, and *suparinpei*) are added through *sandan* by which time practitioners complete the entire curricula). There are other hand, foot, and blocking techniques utilized by *karateka*, of course, but these techniques represent essential components of the *Goju Ryu* martial system. These requirements are phased in gradually throughout the *kyu* ranks. In this manner, *shisochin kata* and *bunkai*, *goshin do ippon kumite*, *kaisai no genri*, and the research paper are the only *new* items required for *shodan* (of course, the required skill level also continues to increase with each advancement).

Basic Techniques

Stances (*Dachi*)
- "L" stance (*renoji dachi*)
- Back stance (*kokutsu dachi*)
- Cat stance (*neko ashi dachi*)
- Crane stance (*hakusura dachi*)
- Cross-foot stance (*bensoku dachi*)
- Formal attention stance (*masubi dachi*)

- Front or forward stance (*zenkutsu dachi*)
- Half-front stance (sometimes called short *zenkutsu*, *shozenkutsu dachi*)
- Hourglass stance (*sanchin dachi*)
- Kneeling (*seiza*)
- Natural stance, feet parallel, (*heiko dachi*)
- Natural stance, toes slightly outward (*hachiji dachi*)
- Side defense stance (*nissin dachi*)
- Side facing horse stance (*kiba dachi*)
- Straddle or sumo stance (*shiko dachi*)

Movement (*tae sabaki waza*)

- Blending
- Evasion
- Moving in stance
- Natural stepping (*ayumi ashi*)
- Shifting/shuffling step *(tsugi ashi)*
- Stance dynamics (balance, stability, strength, weight shifting, distance)
- Turning in stance

Blocking/Receiving (*uke*) Techniques

- "Archer" block (*hara uke*)
- "Mountain" block (*yama uke*)
- Chest block—practiced both open- and closed-hand (*chudan uke*)
- Circular or wheel block (*mawashe uke*)
- Cross block or "X" block (*juji uke*)
- Down block—practiced both open- and closed-hand (*gedan uke*)
- Dropping forearm or wing block (*ude uke*)
- Head block—practiced both open- and closed-hand (*jodan uke*)
- Hooking block (*kakai uke*)

- Inside forearm block (*uchi uke*)
- Press block (*osai uke*)
- Pulling/grasping open-hand block (*hiki uke*)
- Scooping block (*sukui uke*)
- Sweeping block (*harai uke*)
- Wrist block (*koken uke*)

Hand Techniques (*te waza*)
- "Dead arm" strike (*nai wan uchi*)
- Backfist strike (*ura uchi*)
- Double punch (*marote tsuki*)
- Elbow strike (*hiji ate*)
- Finger strike (*nukite uchi*)
- Hammerfist strike (*tetsui uchi*)
- Lunge punch (*oi tsuki*)
- One-knuckle strike (*ippon ken uchi*)
- Palm-heel strike (*shotei uchi*)
- Palm-up center punch (*shita tsuki*)
- Reverse punch (*gyaku tsuki*)
- Standing fist punch (*tate tsuki*)
- Uppercut punch (*age tsuki*)

Leg Techniques (*ashi waza*)
- Back kick (*ushiro geri*)
- Front Kick (*mai geri*)
- Front side kick (*mai yoko geri*)
- Hook kick—inside (*nakanimikazuki geri*)
- Hook kick—outside (*sotomikazuki geri*)
- Joint kick (*kensetsu geri*)
- Knee strike (*hiza ate*)
- Leg block (*ashi uke*)
- Round-house or wheel kick (*mawashi geri*)
- Side kick (*yoko geri*)
- Stomping heel kick (*kakato geri*)

Miscellaneous Techniques
- Breakfall techniques (*ukemi waza*)
- Choking techniques (*shime waza*)
- Combination foot technique drills (e.g., *ashi waza dai ichi*)
- Combination hand technique drills (e.g., *tae waza dai ichi*)
- Focus, power, and control
- Grappling techniques (*katame waza*)
- Joint locking techniques (*kensetsu waza*)
- Throwing techniques (*nage waza*)
- Vital point techniques (*atemi waza*)

Kata & Kata Bunkai
- *Taikyoku kata* (*gedan*, *chudan*, and *jodan*)
- *Gekisai kata dai ichi* and *Gekisai kata dai ichi bunkai*
- *Gekisai kata dai ni* and *Gekisai kata dai ni bunkai*
- *Saifa kata* and *Saifa kata bunkai*
- *Seiyunchin kata* and *Seiyunchin kata bunkai*
- *Saipai kata* and *Saipai kata bunkai*
- *Seisan kata* and *Seisan kata bunkai*
- *Shisochin kata* and *Shisochin kata bunkai*
- *Sanchin kata*
- *Tensho kata*
- Self-defense applications from *kata* (*goshin do ippon kumite*)

Miscellaneous
- Attendance
- Common Japanese words and phrases
- *Dojo* etiquette
- *Dojo Kun*

Appendix A: Hokusei Yudanshakai Advancement Requirements

- First aid and CPR
- Fundamental themes of *Goju Ryu* Karate (strategy and tactics)
- Legal aspects of karate
- Meditation theory and practice
- Methods of instruction
- Research paper
- Stretching theory and practice
- Student evaluation and testing
- Theory of deciphering hidden applications in *kata* (*kaisai no genri*)
- Time in Rank
- Warm-up exercises (*daruma*) theory and practice

APPENDIX B

☀ The Kata of Goju Ryu ☀

Core Kata of Goju Ryu:

Gekisai means "attack and smash, destruction." Created by Chojun Miyagi *Sensei* in 1940 *gekisai* are beginner's *katas*, the first to be learned in some styles. These *katas* introduce the fundamentals of *Goju Ryu* (e.g., stances, attacks, and blocks). *Dai ichi* is the first *gekisai kata* while *dai ni* is the second. The primary difference between the two is the introduction of open-hand techniques and additional stances in *dai ni*.

Saifa means "smash and tear" and is of Chinese origin, brought back to Okinawa by Kanryo Higaonna *Sensei*. It incorporates quick whipping movements and back-fist strikes. *Seiyunchin*, another kata of Chinese origin, means to "pull off balance and fight." *Shiko dachi* (straddle or sumo stance) is emphasized and all of the movements are hand techniques (with no kicks), a distinctive feature.

Goju Ryu relies upon many grabbing and controlling techniques designed to unbalance an attacker and facilitate strikes to vulnerable parts of their body. Translated as "thirteen hands," *Seisan kata* emphasizes this principal with its eight defensive and five offensive techniques. This form stresses close-range fighting with short punches and low kicks to break through an opponent's defenses.

Another *kata* of Chinese origin, *saipai* translates as *"eighteen hands"* (3x6=18). It contains many hidden techniques

149

designed to confuse the opponent in combat. The six represent color, voice, taste, smell, touch, and justice. The three represent good, bad, and peace. *Saipai* has a variety of hand, foot, and body techniques that are somewhat unique within *Goju Ryu kata*.

Shisochin means "battle in four directions", and is sometimes called "four fighting monks." It is rumored to have been one of Chojun Miyagi *Sensei's* favorite *katas* in his later years, well suited to his body. This *kata* is unique to *Goju Ryu* and is not used in other *Naha Te* styles.

Sanseiru means *"thirty-six hands"* (6x6=36), and is sometimes called the "dragon kata." It also focuses on fighting in all four directions. The first six represent eyes, ears, nose, tongue, body, and spirit. The second six represent color, voice, taste, smell, touch, and justice. *Sanseiru* develops low kicks and utilizes many double hand techniques.

Kururunfa is an advanced *kata* featuring *tai sabaki waza* (moving/shifting techniques) and very quick movement. It contains a wide variety of open-hand techniques especially hand and hip coordination techniques.

Sanchin means "three battles." It is a moving meditation designed to unify the mind, body, and spirit. Techniques are done in slow motion such that *karateka* can emphasize precise muscle control, breath control, internal power, and body alignment.

Chojun Miyagi Sensei created *tensho kata*, another moving meditation. *Tensho* means, "revolving hands." It is a combination of hard dynamic tension with deep breathing and soft flowing hand movements, concentrating strength in the *tanden*, and is very characteristic of the *Goju Ryu* style.

Suparinpei represents the number 108 (3x36=108) and has special significance in Buddhism. It is believed that man has

108 evil passions, so in Buddhist temples on December 31, at the stroke of midnight, a bell is rung 108 times to drive away those spirits. The symbolism of 36 is the same as *sanseiru*. *Suparinpai* is *Goju Ryu's* longest *kata*. It utilizes a large number of techniques including breath control and contains the largest number of applicationsfound in any *Goju Ryu kata*.

As an interesting side note, in the 1600s there was supposedly a group of warrior-heroes who had risen above their passions. They traveled the countryside righting wrongs, taking from rich feudal lords, and giving to the poor. This is sort of a Chinese version of Robin Hood and his men. There were said to be 108 of these men, called the 108 hands. Although they were ultimately defeated and scattered, it may have been one of these men who made it to Ryukyu and taught the *suparinpei* form.

Additional Kata:

Taikyoku means, "first course." Gichin Funakoshi *Sensei*, the founder of the *Shotokan* karate style, created the original *taikyoku* series. The *Goju Ryu* versions have been modified to reflect elements within our style, such as the *zenkutsu dachi* (front stance) stances. They all follow the basic H pattern, and increase slightly in difficulty as more techniques are added.

Hookiyu are universal or unified *katas*, created by Seikichi Toguchi *Sensei*, which introduce the basics of *Goju Ryu* stances and defensive postures. They are sometimes considered a simplified form of *gekisai kata*. Some schools teach a third *Gekisai kata* as well.

Gekiha translates as "to destroy something large, very hard, or well fortified." Also created by Seikichi Toguchi *Sensei, gekiha* expands on the basics introduced in *hookiyu* by adding more complex strikes, counter strikes, body movements, and blocks.

Kakuha represents the three basic traditional schools of karate from the three major port cities in Okinawa—*Goju Ryu*,

Shorin Ryu, and *Tomari Te*. It is sometimes translated to represent each school's difference of opinion or separation from each other. It was designed to bring these differences, or representative applications and philosophy, together in one form.

APPENDIX C

Determining Your
✳ Psychological Type ✳

Instructions: Circle the "best" answer for each of the following questions (the answer that best describes you even if it is not entirely accurate). It is best consider your everyday life when answering the questions and not your work life. Record your answers in the table that follows these questions by checking the boxes associated with each of your choices. Count the number of checkmarks in each column to ascertain your most-likely preference for each dichotomy. To validate this conclusion and receive greater depth of understanding about what your personality type means to you, the author suggests that you consult with a professional qualified in the administration of the Myers-Briggs Type Indicator® or, for younger children who are not yet ready for this complex an evaluation, the Murphy-Meisgeier Type Indicator for Children™ (MMTIC™) instrument.

1. *In a social situation I prefer to*
   a. interact with as many people as possible
   b. interact with a few close friends

2. *I am more*
   a. realistic than speculative
   b. speculative than realistic

3. *Which is a greater fault?*
   a. being indiscriminate
   b. being critical

4. *I prefer to work*
   a. to set deadlines
   b. as long as it takes

5. *I prefer*
   a. companionship
   b. solitude

6. *I feel more*
   a. practical then ingenious
   b. ingenious than practical

7. *I am more impressed by*
   a. principles
   b. emotions

8. *I tend to choose*
   a. carefully
   b. impulsively

9. *At parties, I*
   a. stay late and leave
   feeling energized
   b. leave early, feeling
   tired

10. *I am more attracted to*
    a. sensitive people
    b. imaginative people

11. *I am*
    a. hard headed
    b. soft hearted

12. *I am*
    a. punctual
    b. leisurely

13. *Socially, I tend to*
    a. know all the good
    gossip
    b. get behind on the
    "news"

14. *I am more interested in*
    a. what exists today
    b. what is possible
    tomorrow

15. *In judging others, I am
    more swayed by*
    a. laws than circum-
    stances
    b. circumstances than
    laws

16. *It bothers me more
    having things*
    a. incomplete
    b. completed

17. *To relax I prefer to*
    a. visit with friends
    b. read a book

18. *In everyday life, I tend
    to*
    a. do things the usual
    way
    b. do things my own
    way

19. *I am very comfortable
    in making*
    a. logical judgments
    b. value judgments

20. *I prefer things*
    a. settled and decided
    b. unsettled and unde-
    cided

21. *Before I have an important conversation I*
    a. don't worry, just play it by ear
    b. rehearse what I'll say ahead of time

22. *Writers should*
    a. be literal and pithy
    b. express important ideas through analogy

23. *I appreciate*
    a. consistency of thought
    b. harmonious relationships

24. *I am more*
    a. determined and serious
    b. easy going and funny

25. *When giving a speech, I prefer to*
    a. be extemporaneous
    b. prepare carefully ahead of time

26. *Facts*
    a. speak for themselves
    b. illustrate principles

27. *It is worse to be*
    a. unjust
    b. merciless

28. *I usually let events occur*
    a. by careful selection
    b. by chance

29. *I prefer to*
    a. initiate conversation
    b. wait to be approached

30. *Visionaries are*
    a. full of themselves
    b. full of fascinating ideas

31. *I am*
    a. cool-headed
    b. warm-hearted

32. *I feel better about*
    a. having purchased
    b. having the option to buy

33. *New interactions with others*
    a. energize me
    b. tax my reserves

34. *Common sense is*
    a. rarely questionable
    b. frequently questionable

35. *I am more*
    a. firm than gentle
    b. gentle than firm

36. *It is more admirable to be*
    a. organized and methodical
    b. adaptable and flexible

37. *In general I*
    a. enjoy public speaking
    b. do not feel comfortable speaking in front of an audience

38. *As a child I did not*
    a. make myself useful enough
    b. fantasize enough

39. *In making important decisions I prefer to go with*
    a. standards
    b. feelings

40. *I put more value on the*
    a. finite
    b. unlimited

41. *I am*
    a. approachable
    b. reserved

42. *I am more*
    a. practical
    b. fanciful

43. *I am more ruled by*
    a. my head
    b. my heart

44. *I prefer work that is*
    a. contracted
    b. casual

45. *When the phone rings, I*
    a. answer it
    b. hope someone else gets it first

46. *I am more likely to*
    a. see how others are useful
    b. see how others see

47. *I am more satisfied by*
    a. discussing an issue thoroughly
    b. gaining concurrence on an issue

48. *I look for*
    a. familiar patterns
    b. new and interesting things

49. *I prefer*
    a. brief contact with many friends
    b. lengthy contact with few friends

50. *I make decisions based on*
    a. facts
    b. principles

51. *I value being*
    a. unwavering
    b. devoted

52. *I prefer*
    a. a definitive statement
    b. a preliminary statement

53. *In general, I*
    a. speak easily with new acquaintances
    b. find little to say to strangers

54. *I am more interested in*
    a. production and distribution
    b. design and research

55. *To me, the following is a good compliment*
    a. "you are a logical person"
    b. "you are a warm-hearted person"

56. *I feel better*
    a. after making a decision
    b. before making a decision

Answer Sheet for Psychological Type Questions

Record your answer to each question by placing an "X" in the A or B box by each question. Total the number of X's at the bottom of each column. Circle the personality type associated with the highest number in each pair. When all four choices are added together, an estimation of your psychological type will be revealed. To validate this conclusion and receive greater depth of understanding about what your personality type means to you, the author suggests that you consult with a professional qualified in the administration of the Myers-Briggs Type Indicator® instrument. Educators and counselors are often qualified administrators of the instrument. You can also visit the following web sites for more information: www.advisorteam.com, www.keirsey.com, or www.capt.org.

	A	B		A	B		A	B		A	B
1			2			3			4		
5			6			7			8		
9			10			11			12		
13			14			15			16		
17			18			19			20		
21			22			23			24		
25			26			27			28		
29			30			31			32		
33			34			35			36		
37			38			39			40		
41			42			43			44		
45			46			47			48		
49			50			51			52		
53			54			55			56		

E   I   S   N   T   F   J   P

Your scores will show that you have preference for one of the following psychological types (for descriptions of these types, please see page 13):

INFP	ISFP	INTP	ISTP
ENFP	ESFP	ENTP	ESTP
INFJ	ISFJ	INTJ	ISTJ
ENFJ	ESFJ	ENTJ	ESTJ

TABLE 7. PSYCHOLOGICAL TYPE EVALUATION

Here is an example of a completed form:

	A	B
1	X	
5	X	
9	X	
13		X
17		X
21	X	
25	X	
29	X	
33	X	
37	X	
41	X	
45	X	
49		X
53	X	

	A	B
2	X	
6	X	
10		X
14		X
18		X
22		X
26	X	
30		X
34		X
38		X
42	X	
46		X
50		X
54		X

	A	B
3	X	
7	X	
11	X	
15		X
19	X	
23	X	
27	X	
31		X
35	X	
39	X	
43	X	
47	X	
51		X
55	X	

	A	B
4	X	
8	X	
12	X	
16	X	
20	X	
24	X	
28	X	
32		X
36		X
40		X
44	X	
48		X
52	X	
56	X	

11	3

4	10

11	3

10	4

(E) I   S (N)   (T) F   (J) P

Your scores will show that you have preference for one of the following psychological types (for descriptions of these types, please see page 13):

INFP	ISFP	INTP	ISTP
ENFP	ESFP	ENTP	ESTP
INFJ	ISFJ	INTJ	ISTJ
ENFJ	ESFJ	(ENTJ)	ESTJ

TABLE 8. PSYCHOLOGICAL TYPE EVALUATION EXAMPLE

APPENDIX D

❋ Sample Lesson Plan ❋

The following is a sample lesson plan that was developed for teaching *taikyoku kata*. The philosophical concept behind this lesson plan is to build from *kihon* (basic fundamentals) to *kata*, as *taikyoku* is generally taught to entry-level students. We use three versions of this *kata*: *gedan* (done with down blocks), *chudan* (done with chest blocks), and *jodan* (done with head blocks), in ascending order of difficulty. The stance (*zenkutsu dachi*), punches (*oi tsuki*), and basic H pattern are the same for each version. Blocks are simple and done with a closed hand. Punches are all *oi tsuki* (lunge punch) aimed at chin level.

An element of our overall curricula, this *kata* is one of the advancement requirements for *ku kyu* (which does *taikyoku gedan*), *hachi kyu* (which does *Taikyoku Chudan*), and *shichi kyu* (which does *taikyoku jodan*). Higher ranked students need to know it too, of course, but the material will not be new to them.

Although this is a very basic *kata*, really more like a moving drill, it is common to more than one karate system. This commonality and the simplicity of the technique itself make it a straightforward example. Lesson plans for more advanced techniques are more complicated but typically follow a similar approach.

This sample plan could be used for teaching children or adults. For children it may take more class sessions to complete and is generally supplemented with appropriate games and/or competitions to reinforce the learning. I generally limit such activities to no more than 20 percent of the time spent in any class session as they are meant to reinforce rather than present the subject matter. Because games and competitions are discussed in sufficient detail during the body of this work, I have left them out of this example.

Due to the variety of student knowledge levels and prior experience, I have found it more useful to create lesson plans around general subject areas rather than for individual class sessions. This allows more flexibility for adjusting the time required for each component, crossing multiple sessions as necessary. Regardless, assigning time ranges to each component will facilitate organization and enhance an instructor's ability to cover each subject in his or her instructional procedures with an appropriate level of depth. The time ranges in this plan relate to a single training session.

This particular lesson will typically be repeated over a number of class sessions so that students fully understand the *kata*. I intersperse other lesson plans between classes as necessary to maintain interest and motivation levels.

Lesson Plan Section	Comments
Content Students will be able to independently perform Taikyoku kata. Taikyoku chudan will be emphasized.	Content should be derived from core curricula. Taikyoku chudan uses closed-hand chest blocks.
Prerequisites Students must know zenkutsu dachi stance, be able to perform jodan oi tsuki (lunge punch toward head), and chudan uke (closed-hand chest block). Many students will have previously performed this kata but it is not required that they have prior experience with it.	Even if students already know prerequisite techniques, it is a good idea to practice them at least a little prior to performing a new kata. Building from kihon to kata is an effective methodology.
Instructional Objectives Beginning students will understand the pattern of movement, executing stances, blocks, and strikes correctly. Intermediate students will further demonstrate proper pacing, focus, body alignment, and power. Advanced students will apply the concept of "block/control" and develop simple bunkai applications from the kata.	Because most classes are a mix of beginning, intermediate, and advanced students, it is useful to separate educational objectives for each target audience. All skill levels and personality types should derive benefit from each lesson plan (if it is done correctly).
Instructional Procedures 1. Opening ceremony. (5 minutes) 2. Daruma – warm-up, stretch joints, then tendons, then proceed to building muscles. Use zenkutsu dachi as one of the leg stretches during warm-up, emphasizing legs shoulder-width apart (not surfing), both feet facing forward, front leg bent, and back leg straight. Spend enough time on daruma to get everyone thoroughly warmed-up but not so much that they are too tired to learn effectively. (15 minutes)	Timeframes can be altered as necessary during the Plan-Do-Check-Act cycle. Variety in daruma is motivationally important. For great advice on conditioning exercises I recommend www.mattfurey.com. For children, snake push-ups, mountain push-ups or other fun elements should be considered. Daruma should reinforce lesson content where possible.

TABLE 9. LESSON PLAN EXAMPLE

Lesson Plan Section	Comments
Instructional Procedures, continued 3. Kihon – focus on stances, blocks, and punches found in the Kata. Additional techniques from advancement requirements may be added as time permits. (25 minutes)	Building from basics to kata is an effective way to ensure that everyone knows necessary prerequisites. If good progress is not made, adjust time spent in kihon accordingly.
Stances – emphasize moving and turning in zenkutsu dachi. Start with explanation of body alignment, weight progression, and stance dynamics. Demonstrate how to drop to one knee to see that back knee is even with front heel. Show surfing (too narrow) vs. proper stance (shoulder width). Use the following drills to reinforce:	Try to accommodate student predilections by tailoring techniques as appropriate. Be sure to discuss, demonstrate, and practice each technique so that auditory, visual, and kinesthetic modes are addressed.
Tandem drill #1: one partner pushing the other across the room in zenkutsu dachi stance. Tori ("attacker") does a two-hand push in stance while uke ("receiver") offers resisting pressure. Ensure appropriate pressure so that effective body mechanics rather than brute force make the technique successful. Tandem drill #2: one partner moving across the room in zenkutsu dachi while the other holds onto their obi to offer (appropriate) resistance from behind.	When selecting partners, choose students of similar size and weight to the extent practicable. Mix senior and junior students together so that at least one partner has done the drill before and can help ensure that time is used effectively. Use knowledge of student predilections in determining partners when possible as well.
For both drills, have uke step rapidly away or let go of the obi at random moments to check the tori's balance and ensure that it is properly centered.	These drills reinforce proper body mechanics and let students get used to feeling the stance in action. Pressure from behind and from the front help ensure proper balance and stance dynamics.
Blocks – emphasize closed-hand jodan, chudan, and gedan with block/control methodology. Utilize hand shields to strike arms and check for proper alignment and resistance.	Be sure that students understand that most blocks are actually attacks. It is a good idea to have them Kiai on the tenth repetition as they would with a strike.

TABLE 9. LESSON PLAN EXAMPLE *CONTINUED*

Lesson Plan Section	Comments
Instructional Procedures, continued	
Punches – focus on body alignment and hitting with lead knuckle. Utilize striking pads as target.	Kiai on the tenth repetition for punches. If energy level is low, kiai on all punches.
4. Kata – Tie the kihon together with the kata so that connections are obvious (same stances, blocks, and punches; different movement/angles of attack). Step through the movements by count. Go through the entire kata a few times then break it down into component parts, practicing each independently before reintegrating into the whole. Assign goals or focus areas by rank in accordance with instructional objectives (beginning, intermediate, and advanced). (45 minutes)	Sketch the pattern on a white board if available and have senior students demonstrate the kata before the whole class participates. Stagger junior and senior students to facilitate visual learning mode. Freeze students at strategic moments to test body mechanics.
5. Bunkai – Once students have grasped the pattern, explore applications using tandem drills. Allow senior students an opportunity to experiment with what works. Demonstrate possible applications for junior students to employ. Ensure adequate safety by starting slightly out of range and working toward closure. (15 minutes)	Call out kata movements before they are executed the first few times. After several repetitions, have a senior student lead the class a few times so that instructor can watch and correct as required. For bunkai, consider pairing senior students with other seniors rather than with juniors where practicable, as they will get more out of this exercise this way.
6. Kata – Revisit the kata once again keeping bunkai in mind. Ensure that kata movements are not altered. Only mindset and emphasis should change. Follow-up at later class sessions and look for improvement. (10 minutes)	It will likely take more than one class session to achieve instructional objectives. If some students are progressing ahead of others, consider splitting the class.
7. Closing Ceremony. (5 minutes)	After the closing ceremony, I often ask students if they have any final questions before leaving. This is a place to suggest the idea of "homework" practice.

TABLE 9. LESSON PLAN EXAMPLE *CONTINUED*

165

Lesson Plan Section	Comments
Materials or Equipment Needed 1. Open floor space sufficient for number of students taught 2. Hand shield (pads) 3. White board, markers, and eraser (optional, but helpful if available) 4. Mirrored walls (optional, but very helpful if available)	While supplies will generally already be available at the dojo it is a good idea to make sure that everything is in good working order before you need it. Tailor instructional procedures as necessary due to availability of assets (e.g. mirrored walls, space constraints for splitting class, number of instructors, etc.).
Evaluation Process Observe students throughout each step of the instructional procedures. Consider timeframes allotted based on performance: ❑ Kihon should be strong before attempting the Kata. ❑ Basic Kata should be understood before adding Bunkai. ❑ Bunkai must be understood before knowledge of the Kata can be considered adequate. Students should be able to independently perform Taikyoku Kata, working by flow rather than by the instructor's count. Understanding of application should be demonstrated via tandem exercises. Beginning and intermediate students may participate but are not expected to have the same level of execution as advanced practitioners. While one group is testing, the others should watch and try to learn from what they see—emulating the good and avoiding mistakes.	Test beginning students as a group to be sure that they understand the pattern of movement and executing stances, blocks, and strikes correctly. This does not have to be a separate event from the regular instruction. Intermediate students should further demonstrate proper pacing, focus, body alignment, and power. They may be tested with the beginners or separately depending upon personalities of the individuals involved. Test advanced students separately, having them demonstrate bunkai applications with a partner, then describe what they learned to the rest of the class. This will be done as part of the bunkai section.

TABLE 9. LESSON PLAN EXAMPLE *CONTINUED*

Lesson Plan Section	Comments
Follow-Up Activities Assign "homework" to individual students as necessary to reinforce identified strengths or build-up weaknesses in technique or execution.	Unless the same "homework" is given to all students at once, this should be done one-on-one to avoid potentially embarrassing a student.
Instructor Self-Assessment When observing student performance look for common mistakes made by multiple individuals. These areas may represent holes in your instructional approach that need to be addressed.	This is an essential component of the Plan-Do-Check-Act cycle. Instructors should self-assess at every class informally. It is a good idea to document observations monthly and consider revisions of lesson plans as appropriate.

TABLE 9. LESSON PLAN EXAMPLE *CONTINUED*

APPENDIX E

Photograph
✳ Acknowledgments ✳

Chapter 1

A. Tandem moving drills reinforce body mechanics and balance, acclimatizing kinesthetic learners to a stance. Maddie Schenk holds Joey Kane's *obi* as he moves forward in *zenkutsu dachi*. Her pressure should be sufficient to ensure that he has a proper stance without being so strong that Joey has be off-balance to the front in order to move. As he crosses the floor, she will intermittently let go ensure that his balance is adequately centered.

B. Kane *Sensei* demonstrates *saipai kata* while the class watches. Visual learners benefit from watching techniques before attempting do them by themselves. Larry Schenk, Liza Wiberg, Bryan Schenk, Maddie Schenk, and Joey Kane are pictured from left to right in the background.

Chapter 2

C. Weapons forms can add variety to a curriculum, helping with common stances and body mechanics. In this picture Kane *Sensei* and Larry Schenk practice applications from *nicho sai* (two *sai*), a *Matayoshi Kobudo kata*.

D. Maddie Schenk, Bryan Schenk, and Joey Kane run the "Gauntlet of Death," performing techniques on pads/shields held by their instructors. While one can punch or kick the air all day incorrectly with no adverse affect, striking a solid object provides immediate feedback (e.g. if you punch incorrectly, it hurts). Games and competitions help maintain student interest while reinforcing stance, body alignment, movement, and technique.

Chapter 3

E. Students can make dramatic improvements in understanding and technique by teaching and preparing to teach others via role reversal. Maddie Schenk leads the class in *daruma*. The gripping exercise she leads strengthens practitioners' hands and forearms. Repetitions are called in Japanese, affording students an opportunity to practice counting to ten in that language.

Chapter 4

F. Larry Schenk demonstrates an eye gouge with his partner Liza Wiberg. Self-defense applications such as this are inherently dangerous. Participants must be able to trust and respect training partners to fully benefit from such exercises.

G. *Budoka* bow to each other before and after practicing together. This photo represents one variation of an opening or closing ceremony where students, lined-up by rank, bow toward their instructor. Maddie Schenk, Joey Kane, Bryan Schenk, Liza Wiberg, and Larry Schenk are pictured from left or right across from Kane *Sensei*.

H. Franco Sanguinetti *Sensei*, who owns the *dojo* pictured here, has trained under many well-known instructors including Morio Higaonna *Sensei*, Juichi Kokubo *Sensei*, Yoshiaki Gakiya *Sensei*, and Shinpo Matayoshi *Sensei*. Sanguinetti *Sensei* is a *rokudan* (6th degree black belt) in *Goju Ryu* karate and holds rank in other styles such as *Kyokushinkai*, *Shotokan*, and *Shito Ryu*. He has competed in national and international tournaments for thirteen years, and as a result of his experience in competitions, he has earned positions on prestigious teams such as the Peruvian National Karate Team and the Venezuelan National Karate Team. To find out more about Sanguinetti *Sensei* or his *dojo*, please visit www.bushikan.com.

I. Scott Schweizer *Sensei* uses his *tonfa* to block a *bo* strike from Jeff Stevens *Sensei*. Notice how he moves his whole body out of the way. Blunt *kobudo* weapons can cause serious crushing injuries, even death. Extreme vigilance must be used with any weapon practice. Even when solo-training one must always be aware of bystanders and other hazards. Schweizer *Sensei* is a *yodan* (4th degree black belt) in *Goju Ryu* and a *nidan* (2nd degree) in *Matayoshi Kobudo*. He has taught me everything I know about *kobudo*, including how to make the weapons as well as use them. He built both the *tonfa* and *bo* pictured here out of jatoba (Brazilian cherry wood), a very resilient hardwood. Stevens *Sensei* is a *sandan* in *Goju Ryu* karate.

J. Kris Wilder *Sensei* demonstrates *sukui nage* on Jeff Stevens *Sensei*. This technique is common to both judo and karate. Wilder *Sensei* is the owner of the West Seattle Karate Academy as well as its chief instructor. He is a *yodan* (4th degree black belt) in *Goju Ryu* karate, a *nidan* (2nd degree) in Tae Kwon Do, and a *shodan* (1st degree) in Judo. Stevens *Sensei*, another instructor in our *dojo*, is a *sandan* in *Goju Ryu*. Both these gentlemen are exemplary instructors whose example I try to emulate in my own classes. Since each teacher has a unique perspective, I am able to learn more by associating with them collectively than I could with either alone.

K. Scott Schweizer *Sensei* demonstrates a wristlock on Jeff Stevens *Sensei*. While karate focuses primarily on striking techniques it shares locks, throws, and chokes with other art forms such as aikido, jujitsu, and judo. Schweizer *Sensei* is a *yodan* in *Goju Ryu* and a *nidan* in *Matayoshi Kobudo* and is also skilled in aikido. Stevens Sensei is a *sandan* in *Goju Ryu*.

Chapter 5

L. Testing and advancement should be conducted for validation and reinforcement. Here, Larry Schenk strikes Kane *Sensei* in the stomach as he performs *sanchin kata*. *Shime* testing reinforces fundamentals such as concentration, body alignment, movement, and breathing. Kicks, slaps, and punches are firm but never damaging.

M. Kevin Roberts *Sensei* demonstrates *chiishi* techniques. *Nigiri game*, *ishisashi*, *tetsu geta*, *maki* stick, and *makiage kigu* can be seen in the background. A *kyoshi* (master teacher) and 7th degree black belt in *Shorin-Ryu Shorinkan* karate, Roberts *Sensei* operates a *dojo*, personal training business, and a *kigu hojo undo* equipment-manufacturing business. To find out more about *hojo undo* equipment, please visit www.bushifitness.com.

N. Scott Schweizer *Sensei* demonstrates a *chuan no kon*, a *Matayoshi Kobudo bo kata*. Codification of *kata* facilitates a *budoka*'s ability to proficiently and expeditiously learn the art. Schweizer *Sensei* is a *yodan* in *Goju Ryu* and a *nidan* in *Matayoshi Kobudo*.

O. Kane *Sensei* demonstrates the first movement of a traditional *chudan uke* by intercepting Larry Schenk's attack with his forward arm. Once an attack has been fully committed, it can be like trying to catch a bullet to stop it, and so *karateka* are taught to block, check, or deflect as close to the opponent's body as possible as a result of this practice.

P. Once an attack has been neutralized via a block, check, or deflection, *karateka* seize advantage by controlling an opponent with a chambered hand. Kane *Sensei* controls Larry Schenk's arm above the elbow giving forward pressure that entangles the limb long enough to make a counter-attack. Controlling the elbow allows a weaker practitioner to overcome a physically stronger opponent. Notice how open Larry's left side is at this point.

Q. *Seiyunchin kata* utilizes forward moving down blocks. According to the second rule of *kaisai no genri*, what appears to be a block is more properly interpreted as an attack. Pictured from left to right are Larry Schenk, Lawrence Kane, and Liza Wiberg. When teaching *kata* or other moving drills it is important to intersperse senior and junior students so that visual learners can see what is happening in any direction. With only three practitioners, *Sensei* is almost always in the middle.

R. One interpretation of the down block from *seiyunchin kata* is that the practitioner has captured the opponent's arm and is moving forward for a downward strike to the groin, a powerful push-pull technique. The grab is more of a hook such that the thumb is not wrapped around the opponent's wrist. In fighting range, Kane *Sensei's* leg also striking Larry Schenk's knee, breaking his balance. Low stances such as *shiko dachi* are done very close to an opponent because, while quite strong, they are less mobile than other types of stances.

S. When teaching *kumite* to new students, it is a good idea to start slightly out of range. It is essential, however, to help them understand that practical application is much closer. Larry Schenk is pictured with Kane *Sensei* here.

T. Once students understand the movements and have enough control to complete techniques safely, they should begin to practice within fighting ranges. Larry Schenk attacks while Kane *Sensei* demonstrates a more realistic interpretation of the down block from *seiyunchin kata*. Since it is treated as an attack this time, the opponent can be disabled. Note that the elbow and kidneys are struck simultaneously. This movement actually begins with deflection from the right hand immediately followed by an ear slap from the left to disrupt the attacker. In one continuous motion the left hand crosses over the opponent's head and drives down into the elbow/kidney strike. When shown at proper fighting distance, this becomes a substantially more effective technique.

Notes

Introduction and Chapter 1

1. From the book, *Martial Arts Teachers on Teaching* edited by Carol A. Wiley; Berkeley, CA: Frog, Ltd., 1995.

2. *Dojo* means school or training hall and is directly translated as the "place to learn the way." (For those not familiar with Japanese terminology, please refer to the index.)

3. From the book, *Teaching Martial Arts: The Way of the Master* (2nd edition) by Sang H. Kim, Ph.D.; Wetherfield, CT: Turtle Press, 1997.

4. From the book, *Okinawan Goju Ryu II* by Seikichi Toguchi; Santa Clara, CA: Ohara Publications, 2001.

5. Walter Lippmann (1889–1974), author of the nationally syndicated column, *"Today and Tomorrow."*

6. Edward M. Forster (1879–1970), English author and literary critic.

Chapter 2

7. Paladin Associates, a consulting group (www.paladinexec.com/mbti.htm).

8. George Bernard Shaw (1856–1950), playwright and author.

9. Dr. Richard M. Felder, Professor Emeritus of Chemical Engineering at North Carolina State University.

10. Future Now, a consulting group (www.futurenowinc.com).

11. Lau Tzu was a legendary philosopher in the 6th century B.C. Many consider him the father of Taoism.

12. From the book, *Kodokan Judo* by Dr. Jigoro Kano; New York, NY: Kodansha International, Ltd, 1994

13. From the book, *Martial Arts Teachers on Teaching* edited by Carol A. Wiley; Berkeley, CA: Frog, Ltd., 1995.

14. Ibid.

Chapter 3

15. Galileo Galilei (1564–1642), Italian physicist, inventor, and astronomer.

16. From the book, *Okinawan Goju Ryu II* by Seikichi Toguchi; Santa Clara, CA: Ohara Publications, 2001.

17. Ibid.

18. Ibid.

19. "Home Alone: Solo Training Drills Are a Great Supplement to Class Sessions" by Jimmie Nixdorf; *Black Belt Magazine*, September, 1992.

20. From the article, "Goju-Ryu Kenpo" by Chojun Miyagi *Sensei*, a treatise on sanchin *kata*, 1932.

21. From the book, *Okinawan Goju Ryu II* by Seikichi Toguchi; Santa Clara, CA: Ohara Publications, 2001.

Chapter 4

22. Henry David Thoreau (1817–1862), author and transcendentalist.

23. Lawrence Kane, "Introduction to MS Excel" class; Renton Technical College: Renton, Washington.

24. Dr. Inazo Nitobe (1862–1933), a Japanese educator and diplomat whose portrait graces the 5000 yen bank note.

25. From the book, *The Judo Textbook* by Dr. Hayward; Nishioka, Burbank, CA: Ohara Publications, 1979.

26. From the book, *Martial Arts Teachers on Teaching* edited by Carol A. Wiley; Berkeley, CA: Frog, Ltd. 1995.

27. Ibid.

28. Christopher Caile *Sensei*, the founder and editor-in-chief of FightingArts.com.

29. Dave Lowry is a free-lance writer who has trained extensively in the Japanese and Okinawan martial arts. Author of numerous books, he has been the author of a column called "The Karate Way" for *Black Belt Magazine* since 1986.

Chapter 5

30. From the book, *Martial Arts Teachers on Teaching* edited by Carol A. Wiley; Berkeley, CA: Frog, Ltd., 1995.

31. From the book, *The ADHD Solution* by Tom Daly, Ph.D.; San Diego, CA: Smarty Pants Publications 2003.

32. Kris Wilder *Sensei*, (*godan, Goju Ryu* karate; *nidan* tae kwon do; *shodan*, Judo) owner and chief instructor of the West Seattle Karate Academy and author of the book, *Lessons from the Dojo Floor*.

33. Chojun Miyagi *Sensei* (1888–1953), founder of *Goju Ryu* karate.

34. From the book, *Martial Arts Teachers on Teaching* edited by Carol A. Wiley; Berkeley, CA: Frog, Ltd., 1995.

35. Takuda Anshu, an Okinawan Journalist, writing about a karate demonstration by Chojun Miyagi *Sensei*.

36. Morio Higaonna *Sensei*, Chief Instructor of the International Okinawan *Goju Ryu* Karate-Do Federation (IOGKF).

37. From the book, *Martial Arts in America: A Western Approach to Eastern Arts* by Bob Orlando; Berkeley, CA: Frog, Ltd., 1997.

38. Chojun Miyagi *Sensei* (1888-1953), founder of *Goju Ryu* karate.

39. From the book, *Okinawa: Island of Karate* by George W Alexander; Lake Worth, FL: Yamazato Publications, 1991.

40. From the book, *The Truth About Self-Protection* by Massad Ayoob; New York, NY: Bantam Books, 1983.

41. Buddha

42. More specifically, I had a Sig Sauer P220 .45-caliber semi-automatic pistol loaded with MagSafe, +P+ rounds. For readers who are unfamiliar with firearms, MagSafe arguably makes the most effective handgun ammunition in the world. Their pre-fragmented self-defense rounds pretty much guarantee that 1 torso hit = 1 kill because they "explode" upon entry (like being hit by a shotgun from inside your body) causing maximum damage without the danger of over-penetration, which could hit an innocent bystander. The +P+ rounds are so "hot" that they require special springs to control the recoil. At that time I shot competitively on a regular basis, firing nearly 7,500 rounds per year and had extremely good aim. I routinely practiced close-quarter drawing, handgun retention, and stress-fire techniques as well.

43. I generally carry a small amount of cash in my pocket as both a convenience and precautionary measure (rather than simply keeping everything in my wallet). Because my cash was held together with a money clip, I was able to throw the stack of bills a pretty fair distance before running in the opposite direction to escape. The only down side is that the money clip was a present (turquoise inlaid sterling silver) from my parents, which was never recovered. Sure beats having to shoot someone though…

44. From an ESPN interview with "Iron" Mike Tyson, former world heavyweight boxing champion.

45. *"12 Combat Commandments from the School of Hard Knocks"* by W. Hock Hochheim, *Black Belt Magazine*; August, 2003.

46. Washington state law, Revised Code of Washington (RCW) 9A.16.010 definitions.

Chapter 6 and Conclusion

47. Matt Furey is the only non-Chinese gold medalist in Beijing's *Shuai-Chiao* kung fu competition. He is the author of many books including *The Martial Art of Wrestling, Combat Conditioning, Combat Abs*, and *No B.S. Fitness*, which he sells, along with his various videos, at www.matfurey.com.

48. From the Ed Wells Initiative career development web site (http://edwells.web.boeing.com).

49. From the book, *Martial Arts in America: A Western Approach to Eastern Arts* by Bob Orlando; Berkeley, CA: Frog, Ltd., 1997.
50. From the book, *Zen in the Martial Arts* by Joe Hyams; New York, NY: St. Martin's Press, 1979.

Glossary

Romaji (Romanization) note—I have primarily used the *Hebon-Shiki* (Hepburn) method of translating Japanese writing into the English alphabet and determining how best to spell the words (though accent marks have been excluded), as it is generally considered the most useful insofar as pronunciation is concerned. I have italicized foreign terms such that they can be readily differentiated from their English counterparts (e.g., *dan* meaning black belt rank versus Dan, the male familiar name for Daniel). As the Japanese and Chinese languages do not use capitalization, I have only capitalized those words that would be used as proper nouns in English.

Japanese is a challenging language for many English speakers to pronounce correctly. A few hints—for the most part, short vowels are sound just like their English counterparts (e.g., **a** as in f<u>a</u>ther, **e** as in p<u>e</u>n). Long vowels are essentially double-length (e.g., **o** as in <u>oil</u>, in the word *oyo*). The **u** is nearly silent, except where it is an initial syllable (e.g., *uke*). Vowel combination **e** + **i** sounds like d<u>ay</u> (e.g., *bugeisha*), **a** + **i** sounds like al<u>i</u>ve (e.g., *bunkai*), **o** + **u** sounds like fl<u>oa</u>t (e.g., *tou*), and **a** + **e** sounds like l<u>ie</u> (*kamae*). The consonant **r** is pronounced with the tip of the tongue, midway between l and r (e.g., *daruma*). Consonant combination **ts** is pronounced like ca<u>ts</u>, almost a **z** (e.g., *tsuki*).

Arigato gozaimashita
> "thank you for teaching me" said to other practitioners after practicing karate together

budo
> martial ways (arts); sometimes translated as the "martial way of finding enlightenment, self-realization, and understanding"; evolved from *bugei* at the end of the Japanese feudal era, modern *budo* include such arts as judo, karate, aikido, and kendo

budoka
> martial artist, a practitioner of *budo*

bugei
> martial arts, specifically classical martial arts as practiced during the time of the *samurai*

bugeisha
   martial artist, a practitioner of *bugei*

bunkai (or kata bunkai)
   applications or fighting techniques found in *kata*

bunkai oyo
   a series of applications or fighting techniques from a *kata* which have been arranged in a particular flow (logical order)

bushido
   "the way of the warrior," the samurai philosophy, concepts, and ideals that were generally practiced in feudal Japan

chiishi
   stone or concrete

chudan
   chest or middle (for a punch, aim at the solar plexus)

dan
   black belt rank

daruma
   warm-up exercises

dogi (or gi)
   uniform used for practicing martial arts

dojo kun
   precepts or virtues of a *dojo*

dojo
   school or training hall; literally a "place to learn the way"; also called *dojang* in Korean or *kwoon* in Chinese

Dozo one gaishimasu
   "Please teach me" said to other practitioners prior to practicing karate

gedan
   downward (for a punch, aim at the *obi* knot)

gi (or dogi)
   uniform used for practicing martial arts

Goju Ryu
   an Okinawan form of karate developed by Chojun Miyagi *Sensei*, which focuses ~ 70 percent on punching, 20 percent on kicking, 5 percent on throwing, and 5 percent on grappling; literally the "*hard/gentle way of the infinite fist*"

goshin do ippon kumite
   self-defense techniques adapted from *kata*

hanshi
model instructor (someone to be modeled after), generally a senior master instructor of 8th degree black belt or higher who has a specialized certification beyond their rank alone

hikite
a push-pull concept that ensures proper body mechanics for maximum quickness and power in any martial technique

hodoki
unleashing of hands, a trial period for gaining acceptance into a *dojo* in feudal Japan

hojo undo
supplemental training exercises

hyomengi
fighting techniques

ishisashi
a stone padlock, resembling an old-fashioned clothes, iron used for strengthening exercises

itos
first or most important

jari bako
sand box or bowl used for finger thrusts and to condition the hands

jodan
head (for a punch, aim at the chin)

judo
a Japanese martial art developed by Jigoro Kano *Sensei* featuring an emphasis on throwing, grappling, choking, and joint-locking techniques

judoka
judo practitioners (the name of an art form with *ka* on the end refers to it's practitioners)

kaisai no genri
method for deciphering *bunkai* (applications) from *kata*, sometimes called the theory of *kaisai*

kamae
combative posture—standing in *sanchin dachi* (hourglass stance), for example, with one hand in chamber (at the side) and one out in front in a chest block

karate
a (primarily) Japanese or Okinawan martial art which

emphasizes weaponless or empty hand striking techniques (e.g., punching/kicking)

karateka
karate practitioners

kata
a pattern of movements containing a series of logical and practical offensive and defensive techniques

keppan
blood oath sworn upon entrance to a *dojo* in feudal Japan, a loyalty oath signed and sealed with the applicant's blood

kiai
a loud shout or yell to focus one's energy and off-balance an opponent

ki
spirit and energy

kigu undo
supplemental conditioning exercises using various tools or equipment

kihon ido
first basics, a prearranged pattern of basic techniques

kihon
basic or fundamental techniques such as strikes, blocks, or stances

kiso kumite
prearranged sparring using techniques found in *kata*

kiten point
the physical point from which one originated a *kata* (where they were standing when it started)

kobudo
a Japanese or Okinawan martial art featuring a variety of weapons forms

kongoken
heavy rectangular loop used for conditioning

kumite
sparring

Kung Fu
a (primarily) Chinese martial art featuring primarily weaponless or empty hand techniques; literally, "hard work"

kuroi-obi
black belt

kyoshi
> master teaching instructor (teacher of teachers), generally a 6th or 7th degree black belt who has a special certification beyond their rank alone

kyu
> colored belt rank (typically white, yellow, green, blue, or brown)

maki stick
> tuning-fork shaped wooden implement used for conditioning forearms and shins

makiage kigu
> wrist roller used for strengthening exercises

makiwara
> striking post

matayoshi kobudo
> a martial system founded by Matayoshi Shinko *Sensei* which features a wide variety of traditional Okinawan weapon forms such as *bo* (staff), *sai, tonfa, nunchaku, sansetsu* (three-sectional staff), *nunti* (spear), *kama* (sickle), *kuwa* (hoe), *timbe* (hatchet/shield), and *ueku* (oar)

mokuso
> meditation or empty mind

monjin
> person at the gate, someone who had been accepted into the ranks of a *ryu* during feudal Japan

mudansha
> practitioners within the colored belt or *kyu* ranks (*i kyu* or below); literally "no rank"

Naha Te
> a type of karate; empty hand fighting forms indigenous to the *Naha* region of Okinawa

nigiri game
> gripping jars used for conditioning and strength building exercises

obi
> belt

okuden
> hidden teaching, secret techniques of a school or martial style

randori
> free sparring

reishiki
> etiquette or manners

renshi
> senior expert instructor, generally a 5th or 6th degree black belt who has a specialized certification beyond their rank alone

ryu
> system or style of *budo*

sashi ishi
> wooden rod with a weighted ball in the center used for conditioning

sensei
> teacher, literally "one who has come before," a guide to one's development

shihan
> expert instructor, generally a 4th degree black belt or higher who has a specialized certification beyond their rank alone

shimé
> testing for technique and power (usually in relation to *sanchin kata*)

shime waza
> choking techniques

shodan
> first degree black belt; literally "least" or lowest of the *dan* ranks

shogo
> teaching titles or degrees

shomen
> front (of the *dojo*) or place of honor

shugo
> command to line up (at beginning and ending of class) which is usually communicated via a double clap

tan
> wooden log or barbell-like structure used for conditioning

tanden
> center of the body, roughly located at a practitioner's *obi* knot (center of *ki* energy) two finger widths below their naval

tai sabaki waza
> movement, shifting, and evasive maneuvers

tatami mat
> traditional training mat used in judo and other Japanese grappling arts to cushion practitioner's fall and prevent injury; usually 3' x 6'

tatsu
> stand-up; literally to "make straight" or straighten

tetsu geta
> iron clogs used to strengthen kicking techniques

tetsuarei
> dumbbells for weight training

tonfa
> a martial arts weapon, probably originating from a grist mill handle, which is very similar to a modern side-handled police baton

tori
> "attacker" in tandem drills

tou
> bundle of bamboo sticks used for practicing finger strikes

tsuki
> punch, pronounced and sometimes spelled *zuki*

uke
> to receive an attack (block); also the term used to describe the "receiver" in tandem drills (e.g., the one being "attacked")

yanjigo
> a large diagonal step performed after completing a *kata* to return to the place of origination (*kiten* point) and straighten up the line; literally translated as "45 degrees"

yoi
> ready position for beginning a *kata* with hands at waist level, left hand over right, fingers extended together pointing downward

yudansha
> practitioners within the black belt or dan ranks (*shodan* or higher)

Bibliography

Learning styles/Myers-Briggs Type Indicator tool:

Krebs, Sandra Hirsh and Jean M. Kummerow. *Introduction to Type in Organizations*. Palo Alto, CA: Consulting Psychologists Press, Inc., 1990.

Lawrence, Gordon. *People Types and Tiger Stripes: A Practical Guide to Learning Styles*. Gainesville, FL: Center for Applications of Psychological Type, Inc., 1979.

Keirsey, David and Marilyn Bates. *Please Understand Me: Character and Temperament Types*. Del Mar, CA: Prometheus Nemesis Books, 1978.

Teaching and mentoring styles:

Core Concepts for Snowsports Instructors, Des Moines, WA: Professional Ski Instructors of America Education Foundation, 2001.

Strickland, Cindy A. "Differentiated Teaching for Learner Profile." Master's thesis, University of Virginia, 2001.

Wiley, Carol A. *Martial Arts Teachers on Teaching*. Berkeley, CA: Frog, Ltd. 1995.

Graham, Dr. George. *Teaching Children Physical Education: Becoming a Master Teacher (2nd Edition)*. Champaign, IL: Human Kinetics 2001.

Kim, Sang H., Ph.D. *Teaching Martial Arts: The Way of the Master (2nd edition)*. Wetherfield, CT: Turtle Press 1997.

Grasha, Anthony F. and Laurie Richlin. *Teaching With Style: A Practical Guide to Enhancing Learning by Understanding Teaching and Learning Styles*, Pittsburgh, PA: Alliance Publishers, 1996.

Ed Wells Initiative career development web site (http://edwells.web.boeing.com).

Scheyer, Mary, Associate Dean of Business Technology and General Education Programs, Renton Technical College, Renton Washington.

Toastmasters International—leadership and communication training programs.

Martial techniques and instructional methods:

Toguchi, Seikichi. *Okinawan Goju Ryu*. Santa Clara, CA: Black Belt Communications, 1979.

Toguchi, Seikichi. *Okinawan Goju Ryu II*. Santa Clara, CA: Ohara Publications, 2001.

Orlando, Bob. *Martial Arts in America: A Western Approach to Eastern Arts*. Berkeley, CA: Frog, Ltd., 1997.

Nishioka, Hayward. *The Judo Textbook*. Burbank, CA: Ohara Publications, 1979.

Fuller, Joseph's (a.k.a. Sir Caradaugh ap Morgan) medieval combat instruction.

Ito, Hiroo *Sensei's* karate instruction.

Moreland, Robert's (a.k.a. Sir Master Robert' Lancesaisir) medieval combat instruction.

Nishioka, Dr. Hayward *Sensei's* judo instruction.

Rider, Devin *Sensei's* karate instruction.

Sanguinetti, Franco *Sensei's* karate instruction.

Schweizer, Scott *Sensei's* karate and kobudo instruction.

Stevens, Jeff *Sensei's* karate instruction.

Wilder, Kris *Sensei's* karate instruction.

Yamada, Kenji *Sensei's* judo instruction.

Other background research:

Ayoob, Massad. *In the Gravest Extreme: The Role of the Firearm in Personal Protection*. Concord NH: Police Bookshelf, 1980.

Ayoob, Massad. *The Truth About Self-Protection*. New York, NY: Bantam Books, 1983.

The Goju Ryu karate-do web site (www.gojuryu.net).

The Kenshinkan web site (www.kenshinkan.cl).

Franco Sanguinetti *Sensei's* web site (www.bushikan.com).

Index

About the Author

Lawrence Kane has a long history of successful teaching endeavors. As a martial artist, he has taught medieval weapons forms since 1994 and *Goju Ryu* karate since 2002. He developed and presented software application courses at a technical college between 1990 and 1998, where he consistently received student accolades for communicating effectively, demonstrating patience, and fostering a positive learning environment.

Between 1991 and 2000, he was a volunteer mentor and counseled MBA graduates entering the workforce. While mentoring is akin to teaching, there are subtle nuances in the mentor/mentee interaction that make such relationships unique. But just as teaching computers varies slightly from teaching *budo*, the underlying principles of instruction and communication remain the same.

In an effort to enhance business literacy in the aerospace company where he works, he successfully developed and taught the *Decision-Making for Shareholder Value* course, briefed company executives and vice presidents, and presented the *Managing for Value* class to hundreds of employees. As a financial analyst, he has been involved in several unique educational situations where he was tasked with communicating complex financial concepts to non-financial audiences. He routinely delivers management presentations on a variety of business subjects including finance processes, strategic sourcing, and IT infrastructure benchmarking.

Since 1985 he has supervised employees who provide security and oversee fan safety during college and professional football games at a Pac-10 stadium. This part-time job has given him a unique opportunity to appreciate violence in a myriad of forms. Along with his crew, he has witnessed, interceded in, and stopped or prevented literally hundreds of fights, experiencing all manner of aggressive behaviors as well as the escalation process that invariably precedes them. He has also worked closely with the campus police and state patrol officers who are assigned to the stadium and has had ample opportunities to examine crowd control tactics and procedures.

Over the last 30 or so years, he participated in a broad range of martial arts, trying everything from traditional Asian sports such as judo, arnis, kobudo, and karate to recreating medieval European combat with real armor and rattan (wood) weapons. He has also completed seminars in modern gun safety, marksmanship, handgun retention and knife combat techniques, and he has participated in slow-fire pistol and pin shooting competitions. While he certainly claims no mastery in any of the aforementioned activities, he believes that these experiences give him a more diverse viewpoint than the average practitioner of such arts. A well-rounded martial artist, his success in teaching inspired him to write this book as way of sharing his ideas and experiences with others.

Lawrence lives in Seattle with his wife Julie and his son Joey.

COMPLETE BOOK LIST FROM YMAA

6 HEALING MOVEMENTS	B050/906
101 REFLECTIONS ON TAI CHI CHUAN	B041/868
108 INSIGHTS INTO TAI CHI CHUAN—A STRING OF PEARLS	B031/582
ANCIENT CHINESE WEAPONS	B004R/671
ANALYSIS OF SHAOLIN CHIN NA 2ND ED.	B009R/0002
ARTHRITIS RELIEF—CHINESE WAY OF HEALING & PREVENTION	B015R/426
BACK PAIN RELIEF—CHINESE QIGONG FOR HEALING & PREVENTION	B030R/0258
BAGUAZHANG	B020/300
CARDIO KICKBOXING ELITE	B043/922
CHIN NA IN GROUND FIGHTING	B064/663
CHINESE FAST WRESTLING—THE ART OF SAN SHOU KUAI JIAO	B028/493
CHINESE FITNESS—A MIND / BODY APPROACH	B029/37X
CHINESE QIGONG MASSAGE	B016/254
CHINESE TUI NA MASSAGE	B057/043
COMPREHENSIVE APPLICATIONS OF SHAOLIN CHIN NA	B021/36X
COMPLETE CARDIOKICKBOXING	B038/809
EIGHT SIMPLE QIGONG EXERCISES FOR HEALTH, 2ND ED.	B010R/523
ESSENCE OF SHAOLIN WHITE CRANE	B025/353
ESSENCE OF TAIJI QIGONG, 2ND ED.	B014R/639
EXPLORING TAI CHI	B065/424
FIGHTING ARTS	B062/213
HOW TO DEFEND YOURSELF, 2ND ED.	B017R/345
INSIDE TAI CHI	B056/108
KATA AND THE TRANSMISSION OF KNOWLEDGE	B071/0266
LIUHEBAFA FIVE CHARACTER SECRETS	B067/728
MARTIAL ARTS ATHLETE	B033/655
MARTIAL ARTS INSTRUCTION	B072/024X
MARTIAL WAY AND ITS VIRTUES	B066/698
MIND/BODY FITNESS	B042/876
MUGAI RYU	B061/183
NATURAL HEALING WITH QIGONG - THERAPEUTIC QIGONG	B070/0010
NORTHERN SHAOLIN SWORD, 2ND ED.	B006R/85X
OKINAWA'S COMPLETE KARATE SYSTEM—ISSHIN RYU	B044/914
OPENINGS	B026/450
POWER BODY	B037/760
PRINCIPLES OF TRADITIONAL CHINESE MEDICINE	B053/99X
PROFESSIONAL BUDO	B023/319
QIGONG FOR HEALTH & MARTIAL ARTS 2ND ED.	B005R/574
QIGONG FOR LIVING	B058/116
QIGONG FOR TREATING COMMON AILMENTS	B040/701
QIGONG MEDITATION - EMBRYONIC BREATHING	B068/736
QIGONG, THE SECRET OF YOUTH	B012R/841
ROOT OF CHINESE QIGONG, 2ND ED.	B011R/507
SHIHAN TE—THE BUNKAI OF KATA	B055/884
SONG OF A WATER DRAGON	B024/272
TAEKWONDO—ANCIENT WISDOM FOR THE MODERN WARRIOR	B049/930
TAEKWONDO—SPIRIT AND PRACTICE	B059/221
TAO OF BIOENERGETICS	B018/289
TAI CHI BOOK	B032/647
TAI CHI CHUAN	B019R/337
TAI CHI SECRETS OF THE ANCIENT MASTERS	B035/71X
TAI CHI SECRETS OF THE WU & LI STYLES	B051/981
TAI CHI SECRETS OF THE WU STYLE	B054/175
TAI CHI SECRETS OF THE YANG STYLE	B052/094
TAI CHI THEORY & MARTIAL POWER, 2ND ED.	B007R/434
TAI CHI CHUAN MARTIAL APPLICATIONS, 2ND ED.	B008R/442
TAI CHI WALKING	B060/23X
TAIJI CHIN NA	B022/378
TAIJI SWORD, CLASSICAL YANG STYLE	B036/744
TAIJIQUAN, CLASSICAL YANG STYLE	B034/68X
TAIJIQUAN THEORY OF DR. YANG, JWING-MING	B063/432
TRADITIONAL CHINESE HEALTH SECRETS	B046/892
WAY OF KENDO AND KENJITSU	B069/0029
WILD GOOSE QIGONG	B039/787
WISDOM'S WAY	B027/361
WOMAN'S QIGONG GUIDE	B045/833
XINGYIQUAN	B013R/416

COMPLETE VIDEOTAPE LIST FROM YMAA

ADVANCED PRACTICAL CHIN NA - 1	T059/0061
ADVANCED PRACTICAL CHIN NA - 2	T060/007X
ANALYSIS OF SHAOLIN CHIN NA	T004/531
ARTHRITIS RELIEF—THE CHINESE WAY OF HEALING & PREVENTION	T007/558
BACK PAIN RELIEF—CHINESE QIGONG FOR HEALING & PREVENTION	T028/566
CHIN NA IN DEPTH—COURSE 1	T033/086
CHIN NA IN DEPTH—COURSE 2	T034/019
CHIN NA IN DEPTH—COURSE 3	T038/027

more products available from...

YMAA Publication Center, Inc. 楊氏東方文化出版中心

4354 Washington Street Roslindale, MA 02131
1-800-669-8892 • ymaa@aol.com • www.ymaa.com

COMPLETE VIDEOTAPE LIST FROM YMAA (CONTINUED)

CHIN NA IN DEPTH—COURSE 4	T039/035
CHIN NA IN DEPTH—COURSE 5	T040/124
CHIN NA IN DEPTH—COURSE 6	T041/132
CHIN NA IN DEPTH—COURSE 7	T044/965
CHIN NA IN DEPTH—COURSE 8	T045/973
CHIN NA IN DEPTH—COURSE 9	T047/548
CHIN NA IN DEPTH—COURSE 10	T048/556
CHIN NA IN DEPTH—COURSE 11	T051/564
CHIN NA IN DEPTH—COURSE 12	T052/572
CHINESE QIGONG MASSAGE—SELF	T008/327
CHINESE QIGONG MASSAGE—PARTNER	T009/335
COMP. APPLICATIONS OF SHAOLIN CHIN NA 1	T012/386
COMP. APPLICATIONS OF SHAOLIN CHIN NA 2	T013/394
DEFEND YOURSELF 1—UNARMED	T010/343
DEFEND YOURSELF 2—KNIFE	T011/351
EMEI BAGUAZHANG 1	T017/280
EMEI BAGUAZHANG 2	T018/299
EMEI BAGUAZHANG 3	T019/302
EIGHT SIMPLE QIGONG EXERCISES FOR HEALTH 2ND ED.	T005/54X
ESSENCE OF TAIJI QIGONG	T006/238
MUGAI RYU	T050/467
NORTHERN SHAOLIN SWORD—SAN CAI JIAN & ITS APPLICATIONS	T035/051
NORTHERN SHAOLIN SWORD—KUN WU JIAN & ITS APPLICATIONS	T036/06X
NORTHERN SHAOLIN SWORD—QI MEN JIAN & ITS APPLICATIONS	T037/078
QIGONG: 15 MINUTES TO HEALTH	T042/140
SCIENTIFIC FOUNDATION OF CHINESE QIGONG—LECTURE	T029/590
SHAOLIN KUNG FU BASIC TRAINING - 1	T057/0045
SHAOLIN KUNG FU BASIC TRAINING - 2	T058/0053
SHAOLIN LONG FIST KUNG FU—LIEN BU CHUAN	T002/19X
SHAOLIN LONG FIST KUNG FU—GUNG LI CHUAN	T003/203
SHAOLIN LONG FIST KUNG FU—ER LU MAI FU	T014/256
SHAOLIN LONG FIST KUNG FU—SHI ZI TANG	T015/264
SHAOLIN LONG FIST KUNG FU—TWELVE TAN TUI	T043/159
SHAOLIN LONG FIST KUNG FU—XIAO HU YAN	T025/604
SHAOLIN WHITE CRANE GONG FU—BASIC TRAINING 1	T046/440
SHAOLIN WHITE CRANE GONG FU— BASIC TRAINING 2	T049/459
SIMPLIFIED TAI CHI CHUAN—24 & 48	T021/329
SUN STYLE TAIJIQUAN	T022/469
TAI CHI CHUAN & APPLICATIONS—24 & 48	T024/485
TAIJI BALL QIGONG - 1	T054/475
TAIJI BALL QIGONG - 2	T057/483
TAIJI BALL QIGONG - 3	T062/0096
TAIJI BALL QIGONG - 4 MARTIAL APPLICATIONS	T063/010X
TAIJI CHIN NA	T016/408
TAIJI PUSHING HANDS - 1	T055/505
TAIJI PUSHING HANDS - 2	T058/513
TAIJI PUSHING HANDS - 3	T064/0134
TAIJI PUSHING HANDS - 4	T065/0142
TAIJI PUSHING HANDS - 5	T066/0150
TAIJI SABER	T053/491
TAIJI & SHAOLIN STAFF - FUNDAMENTAL TRAINING - 1	T061/0088
TAIJI SWORD, CLASSICAL YANG STYLE	T031/817
TAIJI YIN & YANG SYMBOL STICKING HANDS-YANG TAIJI TRAINING	T056/580
TAIJI YIN & YANG SYMBOL STICKING HANDS-YIN TAIJI TRAINING	T067/0177
TAIJIQUAN, CLASSICAL YANG STYLE	T030/752
WHITE CRANE HARD QIGONG	T026/612
WHITE CRANE SOFT QIGONG	T027/620
WILD GOOSE QIGONG	T032/949
WU STYLE TAIJIQUAN	T023/477
XINGYIQUAN—12 ANIMAL FORM	T020/310
YANG STYLE TAI CHI CHUAN	T001/181

COMPLETE DVD LIST FROM YMAA

ANALYSIS OF SHAOLIN CHIN NA (DVD)	DVD012/0231
CHIN NA INDEPTH COURSES 1 - 4 (DVD)	DVD001/602
CHIN NA INDEPTH COURSES 5 - 8 (DVD)	DVD004/610
CHIN NA INDEPTH COURSES 9 - 12 (DVD)	DVD005/629
EIGHT SIMPLE QIGONG EXERCISES FOR HEALTH (DVD)	DVD008/0037
SHAOLIN KUNG FU FUNDAMENTAL TRAINING - 1&2 (DVD)	DVD009/0207
SHAOLIN LONG FIST KUNG FU - BASIC SEQUENCES (DVD)	DVD007/661
SHAOLIN WHITE CRANE GONG FU BASIC TRAINING 1 & 2	DVD006/599
TAIJIQUAN CLASSICAL YANG STYLE (DVD)	DVD002/645
TAIJI SWORD, CLASSICAL YANG STYLE (DVD)	DVD011/0223
WHITE CRANE HARD & SOFT QIGONG (DVD)	DVD003/637

more products available from...

YMAA Publication Center, Inc. 楊氏東方文化出版中心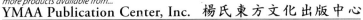

4354 Washington Street Roslindale, MA 02131

1-800-669-8892 • ymaa@aol.com • www.ymaa.com